Endorsements

...*The Second Coming of the White Plague* represents the unique perspective and experience of one of the great figures of modern laboratory medicine, Leonid Heifets. The modern era of TB has been dominated by three transcendent figures: Denis Mitchison, Jacques Grosset, and Leonid Heifets. Heifets has been the conscience of the global TB community. This book should be mandatory reading for all concerned.

- Michael D. Iseman, MD, Professor of Medicine, University of Colorado Health Science Center, Denver, CO

This book is an interesting read with the somewhat unorthodox message that we urgently need a major upgrade in the world's TB laboratory service if we are not to face a massive epidemic of untreatable drug-resistant disease.

- Dennis A. Mitchison, MD Professor, St. George's, University of London, UK

This is an enthralling account of the history of tuberculosis, which relates the enormous strides that have been made in the treatment of this disease. It also tells of missed opportunities with a potentially tragic outcome.

-Amina Jiindani, MD, FRCP
St. Georges, University of London, UK

This book, written by the distinguished TB expert, Professor Leonid Heifets, should be of interest not only to medical professionals, but also to a broad circle of readers. While there are many scientific and popular publications on tuberculosis, many readers will find Leonid Heifets' book both interesting and captivating.

-Michael Perelman, MD
Professor of Surgery, Academician of the Russian Academy of Medical Science Moscow, Russian Federation

Also by Leonid Heifets:

-From Russia with Tales and Confessions to Discovering America, 2009, Dorrance Publishing

- African Exposure, 2010, Tate Publishing

THE SECOND COMING OF THE WHITE PLAGUE

THE SECOND COMING OF THE WHITE PLAGUE

LEONID HEIFETS

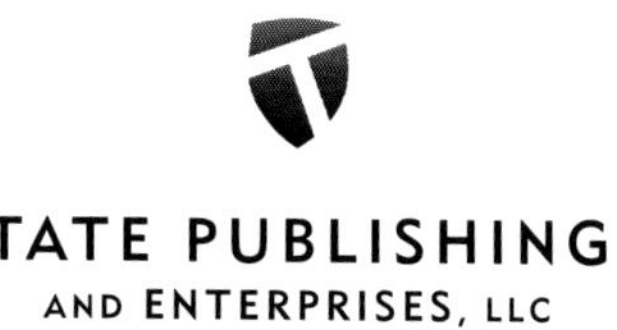
TATE PUBLISHING
AND ENTERPRISES, LLC

The Second Coming of the White Plague

Published by Tate Publishing & Enterprises, LLC
127 E. Trade Center Terrace | Mustang, Oklahoma 73064 USA
1.888.361.9473 | www.tatepublishing.com

Tate Publishing is committed to excellence in the publishing industry. The company reflects the philosophy established by the founders, based on Psalm 68:11,
"The Lord gave the word and great was the company of those who published it."

Cover design by Allen Jomoc
Interior design by Jomel Pepito

Published in the United States of America

ISBN: 978-1-62147-875-1
1. Medical / Infectious Diseases
2. Medical / Public Health
12.11.23

Dedication

In memory of the millions of people dying of tuberculosis in our time.

To the medical professionals around the world who are making valiant attempts to stop this modern plague!

Table of Contents

Foreword

It is a great pleasure for me to write the foreword for the present book written by my friend and colleague, Leonid Heifets. Like me, Leonid suffered from tuberculosis, was a medical doctor and a microbiologist, and devoted a great part of his life to combat our common adversary: the tubercle bacillus. Together, we are zealots in the quest for eradication of tuberculosis. If this explains the background of the book, it does not tell the reader why he or she should absolutely read it.

The book should be read because it is well written and scientifically accurate. It pays tribute to the decisive role of the scientists who have paved the way for the control of tuberculosis and explains clearly what has been achieved and what remains to be achieved to prevent a deadly resurgence of the white plague, this time resistant to antibiotics. Yet beyond this essential information, the real reason to read Leonid's book is rooted in its unconventional, often impertinent and politically incorrect presentation. Of course, Leonid settles the score with the bureaucrats of all sides, his "usual suspects." But, in depth, the book is not at all polemical in nature; rather it is a mixing of personal anecdotes and scientific matters to ensure that its readers, especially those who are not specialists, understand the gravity of the current challenges of global efforts to control tuberculosis.

We find ourselves at a critical moment in the history of tuberculosis, despite the ancient nature of this disease. The successful treatment and control of tuberculosis rests entirely on the translation of scientific discovery into stringent implementation of control measures. Leonid's discussion of the significance of the laboratory setting as the heart of the eradication mission is presented with eloquence and accuracy. His writing is a history of the path to our present circumstance and yet, no less a call to arms for our continued fight, most importantly in the many nations where tuberculosis remains an avoidable, unjustified, and preventable epidemic. Leonid reminds us that to succeed in our fight against the tubercle bacillus we must also overcome the obstacles created by our inaction, scientifically and politically. If we continue to fail to fulfill our promise to do everything in our power to stop tuberculosis, then I assure you Leonid's next book will be a history of how we missed our chance to do what we already knew we could and should. I hope you enjoy reading his book as much as I have, and I hope too that it will open your eyes and motivate you to take action.

- Jacques Grosset, MD
Johns Hopkins University
Center for TB Research

Preface

For many years the general public erroneously viewed tuberculosis as a problem of the past. It is recognized today that tuberculosis is one of the most alarming health problems in the world, with almost two million people dying from this illness every year. The purpose of this book is to present information indicating that the current spread of drug-resistant tuberculosis across the globe may lead to epidemics of incurable forms of this disease.

It sounds an alarm about this critical situation and about insufficient current control measures to prevent this from happening. The book also addresses the measures that should be taken to diminish probable epidemics of incurable disease. To paint a comprehensive picture of the problem, the book also reviews the history of tuberculosis, in conjunction with the past, present, and possible future of tuberculosis research.

The book is addressed not only to the broad audience of medical professionals and those who are not involved with tuberculosis, but also to the general public. It is a difficult task to explain some complex medical issues in simple terms. For the benefit of potential readers with only limited knowledge of tuberculosis, the book is divided into two parts.

Part 1 is a short summary of current basic knowledge about this infectious disease. It takes into account such issues as current perceptions of tuberculosis by the media and the public at-large, history of the disease, and major scientific discoveries in the field.

Part 2 presents the worldwide problem of drug-resistant tuberculosis, including analyses of the causes of such epidemics and measures necessary to prevent them. One of the aims of Part 2 is to educate the public on the threat of epidemics of incurable tuberculosis due to the spread of drug-resistant forms of the disease, particularly of the multi-drug resistant tuberculosis (MDR-TB).

It is impossible to not use some medical and public health terms in describing the situation and in statements related to the measures necessary to prevent these epidemics. Professional terminology, and some abbreviations or acronyms are commonly used to describe the current situation in the world and the future trends of the tuberculosis epidemics.

Some of these terms are introduced in the text, but a complete reference list of terms is presented in Appendix 1.

The essential statistical data and other factual material have deliberately been excluded from the text to provide easier reading. These materials can be found in Appendices 2-6.

Introduction: The Anti-Tuberculosis Manifesto

A specter is haunting the world—the specter of a new white plague, the specter of incurable tuberculosis epidemics. The term *white plague* was used to describe the tuberculosis epidemic that killed about 25 percent of the Europeans in the nineteenth century. Today tuberculosis is almost 100 percent curable, but that may change. According to the numerous publications by the World Health Organization, tuberculosis (TB) takes the life of another human being every twenty seconds, and worldwide TB kills almost two million people each year, more than the number of deaths from AIDS, malaria, and leprosy combined. TB is an infectious disease, and most threatening is the growing spread of drug-resistant tuberculosis. This occurs when patients are not responding to therapy with the commonly used anti-tuberculosis drugs and infecting others with these dangerous bacteria. A specter is haunting the world.

Tuberculosis is predominantly a lung disease, but other organs may be involved as well. In severe cases a person becomes emaciated, which is the reason TB became known as a wasting disease or consumption. Besides weight loss, other symptoms typical of TB are: fever, cough, and night sweats. TB can appear in a generalized (disseminated) form affecting all systems of the body, occurring mainly in individuals with deficient immunity, in particular persons who are infected with HIV.

The germs causing tuberculosis (tubercle bacilli) were discovered in 1882, but no cure was known at that time. Sixty to seventy years later, after the discovery of the first anti-tuberculosis drugs in the 1940s, hopes were high that tuberculosis epidemics would no longer affect mankind. Contrary to these expectations, tuberculosis became the world's most neglected health problem during the second half of the twentieth century, resulting in a growing number of TB patients and high death rates in many countries.

The neglect was mainly due to failure to adjust control measures in tuberculosis epidemics in developing countries to specific situations in given locations. Moreover, a significant part of the problem became a political issue, often more so than a medical problem.

The situation became especially severe during the last three decades due to a number of new problems. One was the growing number of individuals with HIV/AIDS who are highly vulnerable to tuberculosis, which is often difficult to diagnose in these cases due to increased possibility of unusual clinical manifestation of TB in these individuals. The growing dual TB+HIV epidemic created a new dangerous reservoir of TB infection enhanced by the epidemic of drug abuse. Often, the interconnected epidemics of HIV and TB stem from an epidemic of drug-related crimes, when the infected individuals are concentrated in prisons, ultimately resulting in a high level of transmission of HIV and TB in prisons.

Another major current problem is the growing prevalence of drug-resistant tuberculosis. Initially it was the result of uncontrolled administration of TB drugs and non-compliance of patients with the prescribed treatment regimens. Denial of the problem and failure to address it in a timely manner and in a reasonable non-political fashion, resulted in growing rates of multi-drug resistant (MDR), and recently, in extensively drug-resistant (XDR) tuberculosis.

MDR is defined as resistance of the tubercle bacilli to at least two most important drugs: rifampin (RMP) and isoniazid (INH). XDR is defined as resistance not only to RMP and INH, but also resistant to one of the injectable drugs (amikacin, kanamycin, capreomycin) and to the potent new drugs belonging to a class of quinolones (ofloxacin, levofloxacin, moxifloxacin). These types of resistance leave very few choices of therapy for the treating physician.

Most cases of TB in the US, including cases of drug-resistant tuberculosis, are related to the "importation phenomenon," tuberculosis among the foreign-born individuals. Particular attention should have been given to the possibility of infection from non-immigrant visitors having unidentified TB, which should alarm the public health officials (the system does address testing of the legal immigrants). It is clear that the US is not isolated from the rest of the world when it comes to the spread of any infection.

The specific tuberculosis problems in the US has been addressed in many publications, including numerous documents issued by the Center for Diseases Control and Prevention (CDC), but the problem of possible *importation* of tuberculosis by non-immigrant visitors and the possibility of testing them for TB before their arrival to the US has not yet been properly acknowledged.

The growing rates of highly drug-resistant incurable tuberculosis in some areas of the world may reach the level of a new *white plague* despite the efforts by the World Health Organization (WHO) and many other governmental and nongovernmental organizations and groups, including very significant financial support from the US and other countries. In view of general availability of at least twelve drugs to treat TB (not all are readily available in some specific areas of the world), the situation is puzzling, triggering many questions such as: Is anything wrong with the current international policies and many national TB control programs? What is the significance of inconsistency in policies of these organizations? How should the priorities among the urgently needed measures be selected? What can and should be done in the short term, and what would be a long-term approach?

There is not enough awareness among medical professionals and the general public concerning the fact that the world is on the brink of epidemics of incurable TB, and that tuberculosis is already a major world problem that affects social life and economics of the whole world. Along with insufficient information targeting public attention, politics play a significant role in the failure of international organizations to implement effective tuberculosis control measures. It is important that concerned people and organizations sound the alarm concerning this real and present danger. Again, a specter is haunting the world—the specter of a new white plague.

Part 1

Tuberculosis: A Social and Historic Perspective

Staged Publicity and the Fate of Individuals

For the first time, media attention to the problem of tuberculosis was triggered during the seven outbreaks of the disease in 1980s and 1900s in New York City and Florida, with more than 90 percent mortality among approximately 200 patients (mostly prisoners), many of whom were also infected with HIV. Attention of the media to the problem at that time called for appropriate actions of the officials and society that significantly helped to reverse the situation.

In 1993, the famous journalist Deborah Norville created a TV program for the NBC newsmagazine called *Street Stories* that focused on the tuberculosis problem. I had the honor of being interviewed by this most intelligent woman.

Her first question was, "How can one become infected with TB; how is this infection spread?"

My answer was simple: "TB patients may produce small droplets of fluid into the air when coughing or sneezing, and even while talking and laughing. People around them are exposed to the TB infection if these droplets contain tubercle bacilli."

The next question was much more serious: "If that is so, do you think that a TB patient whom I met at your hospital a while ago, and who came to Denver by airplane, could endanger a passenger who was sitting next to him in the aircraft?"

My answer was, "No, not only the passenger next to him, but everybody in the airplane, because most of the air in any aircraft is circulating without any substantial filtration."

Along with a story about my involvement, the presentation included interviews with Drs. Lee Reichman, William Stead, and Edward Nardell. These experts expressed their opinion that TB is not very infectious.

Dr. Reichman said, "If you are not coughing, you cannot spread the infection." Among other stories on this show was a presentation about an outbreak of TB in the small town of Bath, Maine where a person with laryngeal TB (when TB is affecting the vocal cord) settled in Bath and infected many people. This form of tuberculosis makes the patient very contagious. At least twenty-one cases of active TB occurred between 1989 and 1992 among those who had direct contact with this patient, followed by a number of secondary cases.

The *Street Story* by Norville was the first time the media addressed the problem of drug-resistant TB and the issue of the dual TB+HIV infection. It also demonstrated the controversy in opinions among the experts regarding the infectiousness of people with TB.

The real life cases described below demonstrate inconsistency in many reports by the media: on one hand, sensationalism around some individual cases, and on the other, insufficient attention given to the danger of epidemics of drug-resistant TB globally. These stories also highlight inconsistency in the medical authorities approach to the issue of traveling of some TB patients.

Mr. Andrew Speaker's story(1)

At the time of this writing Mr. Andrew Speaker has fully recovered from his bout with tuberculosis, which did not significantly affect his health. However, his life was torn apart and his reputation was ruined by the political issues that surrounded his case, and by the relentless attention he received as a TB patient by society, medical authorities, and the media. He was often portrayed as a public enemy, spreading dangerous tubercle bacilli around the world and by doing so, endangering the lives of many. He was even the subject of a Federal Isolation Order issued for the first time in more than forty years, by the CDC.

In March of 2007, Mr. Speaker developed pain in the left side of his chest and was diagnosed with tuberculosis after a chest X-ray revealed a typical lesion. He did not have the usual symptoms of TB such as fever, night sweats, and coughing. However, because of pain in his left ribcage, his physician ordered a chest X-ray. Since he was not coughing and could not produce any phlegm (sputum), a bronchoscopy procedure was performed to obtain a specimen directly from his bronchi for laboratory examination. This examination confirmed that Mr. Speaker had active tuberculosis and that his tubercle bacilli were resistant to the two main anti-tuberculosis drugs: rifampin (RMP) and isoniazid (INH).

According to current classification of this illness, resistance to these two drugs is a basis for diagnosis of multi drug-resistant tuberculosis (MDR-TB). Subsequently, resistance to two more drugs (ethambutol and pyrazinamide) was discovered, and treatment with these four drugs was stopped. Testing (by a quite a sophisticated procedure called sequencing of the DNA of the bacteria) in the CDC laboratory on May 9 did not detect resistance to other drugs, which meant that he did not have "extensively drug-resistant tuberculosis" (XDR-TB).

Mr. Speaker told me that on May 10, 2007 his local physicians and epidemiologist where he lived suggested that he should travel to the National Jewish Health in Denver for consultation where the physicians are more experienced in the proper treatment of his form of tuberculosis. In addition, they explained to Mr. Speaker that he was not contagious and did not represent any threat to others, because he did not have a cough and the microscopic examination of his bronchial washings smear specimen did not reveal any tubercle bacilli. Usually, negative sputum smear microscopy results mean that the tuberculosis patient produces only small number of tubercle bacilli that can be detected only by methods other than microscopy.

Since Mr. Speaker was getting married, he suggested to his physician that he would go to Denver for consultation on the way back from his honeymoon. His physician did not object to this plan. On May 12, Mr. Speaker travelled to Paris, and then to Greece where the wedding ceremony took place, followed by a honeymoon in Italy.Mr. Speaker's father-in-law, Dr. Cooksey, an employee at CDC, returned from the wedding ceremony in Greece on May 22 to Atlanta and learned that the Mr. Speaker's diagnosis at CDC was changed from MDR-TB to XDR-TB (extensively drug-resistant tuberculosis). The CDC based this change on some new laboratory test results that indicated drug resistance to a new class of drugs called quinolones and to some injectable drugs, in addition to resistance to RMP and INH. After Mr. Speaker learned of the new development from Dr. Cooksey, he contacted the CDC and was told by the CDC representative that he should turn himself over to Italian medical authorities for quarantine and treatment, which he was told would take nearly two years. Instead, Mr. Speaker decided to cut-short his honeymoon and travel to the US for proper treatment by expert physicians as previously recommended. Regardless of the change in diagnosis, Mr. Speaker still did not cough and did not produce sputum, which he perceived as an indication that he was still not contagious.

Apparently, Mr. Speaker's case presented the opportunity to demonstrate the vigorous stand of the CDC in protecting the public from *irresponsible behavior* by individuals who fail to obey orders issued by the CDC. Unprecedented measures were taken to apprehend and quarantine Mr. Speaker upon his return to the US and, for the first time in more than forty years, the CDC issued a Federal Isolation Order. The CDC and the media reported on the case (without Mr. Speaker's consent), and a website appeared condemning the *irresponsible* person who was spreading very dangerous TB bacteria around the world.

Upon his arrival in the US on May 25 Mr. Speaker immediately checked into the Bellevue Hospital in New York, and notified the CDC of his arrival. He was eventually transferred to National Jewish Health in Denver. Our laboratory received and retested the TB cultures that had been isolated and tested by the CDC. On June 10, 2007, I reported the results of our testing at National Jewish, which indicated that the tubercle bacilli from Mr. Speaker were resistant to rifampin, isoniazid, and pyrazinamide, but fully susceptible to all quinolones and to all injectable drugs. That meant that Mr. Speaker did not have XDR, but only MDR, as originally diagnosed.

The CDC laboratory accepted our statement, and subsequently reported the same results showing that the culture from Mr. Speaker was not resistant to quinolones and second-line injectable drugs (amikacin, kanamycin, capreomycin). The CDC laboratory used only one technology for drug susceptibility testing—the agar-proportion method. In addition to the agar proportion method, our laboratory used a more sophisticated quantitative method in a liquid culture medium. The latter is a rapid test providing results in a shorter period of time than the agar proportion method. Our final results were reported sooner than those by CDC and the Bellevue Hospital in New York. Results by both methods for all cultures (from CDC and New York, and cultures isolated in our lab) were identical, which confirmed the validity of the test results reported by us.

The CDC did not admit any error or mistake in the previous report, either technical or clerical, although CDC director, Dr. Julie Gerberding, testified before the Senate Committee stating that there had been several mistakes. CDC representatives suggested that the difference between results at CDC and National Jewish could be because the National Jewish laboratory used an experimental method (referring to the test in the liquid medium). In fact, this method (in addition to the same test as in CDC) has been in use for more than twenty years, and has been described in detail in many publications.

Also, CDC representatives suggested that Mr. Speaker had two sub-strains of tubercle bacilli, and perhaps the initial report of XDR from CDC was related to one of these strains representing XDR bacteria in the specimen. Furthermore, CDC stated that this original XDR isolate was "not available anymore." (What that meant is not clear—mysteriously dead? Destroyed?) Some experts, being concerned with the CDC's reputation, publicly supported the idea that the CDC test actually detected a small portion of the

XDR strain. We tested three specimens, including the culture isolated at CDC, as well as material removed from Mr. Speaker's lung during surgery, and could not verify the hypothesis that he had different sub-strains with different drug-susceptibility patterns. While such findings are possible, particularly in patients with multiple lesions, this was not the case with Mr. Speaker, who had only one lesion in his lungs.

In her article in *The Atlanta Journal-Constitution* (January 13, 2008), Alison Young (2) criticized the actions of the CDC in dealing with the Mr. Speaker's case, and referred to interviews with top experts in the field (Drs. Iseman, Burman, and Reichman) stating that Mr. Speaker was at a very low risk of causing transmission. She criticized the actions of the CDC as staging publicity for purely political reasons and to justify requests for additional funds from the government.

In Denver, Mr. Speaker received vigorous treatment with antibiotics selected on the basis of expedited laboratory testing with fourteen drugs against his bacteria. In addition, the TB lesion in his left lung was surgically removed on June 17, which expedited his successful recovery. There was a question as to whether he would have received equivalent expedited testing and treatment at the hospital in Italy.

The personal life of this individual was in shambles, but not from tuberculosis. He fully recovered from the illness, but his personal and professional reputation was destroyed by the public campaign waged against him. People neither noticed, nor did they pay attention to the corrected CDC report, but rather remembered Mr.

Speaker as a kind of a public enemy, an irresponsible person spreading dangerous TB bacteria. Aside from the fact that his personal life was ruined, this incident also resulted in the loss of his business.

The CDC used the case of Mr. Speaker to demonstrate the vigilance of this organization in protecting the interests of the public, and CDC officials often referred to the manuals and regulations restricting known TB patients from traveling by air. Obviously, there are no instruments to control this from happening when the traveler is not identified as a TB patient. Moreover, the rules related to the air travel of the known TB patients can be *modified* by the CDC when politically necessary. For example, a child, diagnosed with multi-drug resistant tuberculosis, adopted by American parents, was recently (in 2011) allowed to travel with special CDC permit on a passenger aircraft from China to the US. Apparently, the primary reason for the CDC's different approach in this case was influenced by involvement of the Chinese government.

Refusal to grant such a permit may have had some negative publicity and political consequences. Perhaps, the permit to travel in this case of the diagnosed MDR-TB was based on "exceptional circumstances" as it is worded in the *WHO 2008* document "Tuberculosis and Air Travel." (3) There are guidelines for travel restrictions by WHO and CDC, and there are many quite complex situations when a TB patient can be removed from the *Do Not Board* (DNB) list, but the fact is that different approaches are possible to the issue of travel of the known TB patients, and the differences are often motivated more so by politics than by issues of health or safety.

Mrs. A's story

I met Mrs. A. twice, once upon her arrival to the US and before her departure back to her home country. She came to the US as a tourist having highly contagious tuberculosis. Her sputum contained millions of tubercle bacilli that were resistant to most of the drugs. She could not receive proper treatment in her country, but she was fortunate to be a member of a very wealthy family. She came to the US as a tourist, checked in to the best hospital, and paid a fortune in cash for her hospitalization and treatment. This case is not unique, but condemnation of such individuals similar to those that targeted Mr. Speaker was neither expressed by the CDC, nor by society.

Mr. Juarez's story

An example of a story completely different from that of Mr. Speaker's was a publicity-motivated article by Margie Mason and Martha Mendoza published by the Associated Press (AP) on December 27, 2009 titled, "First Case of Highly Drug-Resistant TB Found in US." It is a story of a nineteen-year-old man who came from Peru as a student to the US. This article was publicized through the internet and by a number of press agencies. There are a few problems with this article and its publicity. First, the statement in the title is not accurate because the case described was not the first case of highly resistant TB in the US. In fact, a number of cases of MDR or XDR have been reported in the US annually since 1993, resulting (as reported by CDC) in a total of 2,927 cases of MDR and forty-nine cases of XDR (4).

Secondly, according to the report, Mr. Oswaldo Juarez was successfully treated to full recovery at the A. G. Holley State Hospital in Florida. This success would not have been possible if the tubercle bacilli were resistant to all anti-tuberculosis drugs, leaving no choice for treatment. New anti-tuberculosis drugs, namely quinolones (for example, moxifloxacin and levofloxacin) and linezolid were not available in Peru yet, and therefore no tubercle bacilli resistant to these drugs could have been circulating in there.

Therefore, it is most likely the bacteria that caused TB in Mr. Juarez were susceptible to these drugs. It is unfortunate that the authors of the article failed to mention it, as well as any specifics for their definition for XDR in this case, or which drugs were used for patient's therapy. The fact that the patient's bacteria were susceptible to the quinolones would disqualify definition of the strain/isolate as XDR. Most likely, the isolate was resistant only to the so-called first-line drugs, such as RMP and INH, resulting in resistance to these commonly used around the world agents.

Such data could have been the basis for definition of MDR, but not XDR. Unfortunately, not satisfied with the erroneous claim that the patient had XDR, the authors of the article introduced two new acronyms—

XXDR and CDR (completely drug-resistant). Introduction of this new terminology is unjustified and may only cause more confusion. The case described in the article definitely represented a challenge to physicians because of a very limited choice of drugs for treatment. According to the article, the treatment leading to the recovery lasted for nineteen months and cost $500,000 to the Florida taxpayers.

The situation with emergence of drug resistant TB cases and their importation to the US is very serious, and there is no need for it to be sensationalized. Moreover, it may have a reverse effect, especially when based on inaccurate information. At the same time, the authors missed the opportunity to emphasize that it was an example of an *imported* case, as Mr. Juarez came to the US from Peru as a visiting student. He was not checked for TB at arrival, and the diagnosis of TB was surprising for him, as well as for the medical authorities. The authors mentioned that millions of visitors are coming to the US unchecked for TB, and that 82 percent of the new TB cases identified in 2007 were among foreign–born individuals. At the same time, they did not make an emphasis that the described case is a definite call for measures to prevent importation of drug-resistant tuberculosis to the US. They could have used this situation to stress the need for enhanced measures to diminish the frequency of such occurrences, regardless of the patient's level of drug resistance of bacteria.

Mr. Robert Daniels' story

Sara Gandy posted the story about Robert online (5, 6). I met Robert on July 27, 2007 while he was hospitalized at National Jewish Health in Denver. Here is his story as he (7) told me, along with information from Sara Gandy's articles.

He was born in Moscow. His parents divorced, after which his father immigrated to the US. At age eleven, Robert joined his father in Arizona, and at the age fourteen, he received dual US-Russia citizenship. Back in Moscow at age seventeen, he did not finish school, and later became involved in minor crimes, which resulted in his imprisonment. During his short (less than a year) stay in jail, he contracted TB. He was treated in the prison hospital, and later at the local Russian TB dispensary.

After learning a life-lesson, he changed his lifestyle, got married, and started a family. He has a son, who was six years old at the time I spoke to him. In 2006, Robert realized that his TB worsened despite continued treatment at the Russian dispensary with four medications. At age twenty-six, he decided to move to the US in search of better treatment and came to Phoenix, Arizona. At the beginning of 2007, he received therapy for his illness, which was diagnosed as drug-resistant tuberculosis. As in Mr. Speaker's case described above, he was diagnosed with XDR-TB, which was later changed to MDR-TB in Denver.

He was arrested for appearing in public without a mask when he went for a walk upon his return to

Arizona. The judge ruled that he exposed others to the danger of being infected with tuberculosis. According to the article by Sara Gandy, Mr. Daniels became the *special attention* target of Maricopa County Sheriff, Joe Arpaio. In jail, Robert was placed in isolation and under video surveillance and was deprived of standard comforts as a prisoner. After complaints, including the involvement of the American Civil Liberties Union, Mr. Daniels was allowed to travel to Denver, where he received appropriate therapy, including surgical intervention.

Intensive testing was performed in our laboratory, and we found that his tubercle bacilli were resistant to three drugs he received in Russia (isoniazid, rifampin, and streptomycin). This data justified the definition of MDR, but not XDR as previously determined in Arizona. His bacteria were susceptible to many agents, which provided our physicians with several choices for effective therapy. In September, after significant improvement of his condition, Robert was allowed to go back to Arizona, but was fearful of the sheriff who had threatened to place him back in jail. Shortly after his return to Arizona, he quickly returned to Moscow to avoid the possible harassment from the sheriff and to join his family.

In summary: About TB Importation

The stories above illustrate either compliance or noncompliance with the existing regulations. In reality there are obvious inconsistencies in the approach of public health authorities in dealing with travel restrictions of different TB patients. On one hand, no restrictions had been applied to Mrs. A and the adopted child from China. On the other hand, excessive publicity was given to the cases of Mr. Speaker, Mr. Juarez, and Mr. Daniels; all three had MDR-TB but were initially misdiagnosed as cases of XDR-TB.

We should stress that regardless of the differences in combinations of antibiotics selected for treating patients with XDR vs. MDR, there is no difference between them in the level of possibly transmitting the infection to others. In reality, patients with both types of illness represent a great danger in spreading an epidemic of drug-resistant tuberculosis. At the same time, an accurate diagnosis (MDR vs. XDR) is important for both accurate public knowledge and proper therapy.

In all three cases mentioned above, the misdiagnosis of XDR was based on preliminary testing, each time by only one laboratory method. It is essential that such a serious diagnosis as XDR be based on confirmation by at least two different methods, and to be repeated in case of discrepancy in results reported by different laboratories.

There are documents issued by the WHO and CDC regulating and restraining air travel of the TB patients: WHO, Tuberculosis and Air Travel, Geneva, Second edition, 2006 and Third edition, 2008; and CDC, Federal Air Travel Restrictions (8). According to these documents, all infectious and potentially infectious TB patients must not travel on commercial flights until their sputum becomes smear-negative after appropriate therapy. Likewise, patients with MDR-TB and XDR-TB must not travel until two negative sputum and cultures are obtained. The problem is that these well-written and detailed documents apply to already identified TB patients when it is known that they intend to travel. These or any other publications do not address the issue of detecting TB in unidentified TB patients (diagnosed and not diagnosed) who intend to travel.

There are thousands of highly infectious TB patients producing smear-positive sputum—which is an indication of a high content of bacteria—traveling throughout the world, some of them with MDR or XDR. An unknown number of them are coming to the US, and most of the new cases of tuberculosis in this country are related, directly or indirectly, to importation.

The role of importation of TB from one country to another is not universally recognized. For example, most recently the AP referred to a report (9) entitled "London, Tuberculosis Capital of Western Europe." It stated that in 2009 the number of TB cases in London increased to 3,540 cases during the last decade, with even incomplete data of up to 9,000 cases in Britain, with rates (15 per 100,000 population) higher than in the rest of Europe.

The article stated that most of these cases are in people born overseas, although not in recent arrivals, and that 85 percent of them were in Britain for more than two years. The author of this commentary, Dr. Alimuddin Zumla, of University College London, stated that the rise in tuberculosis has nothing to do with migration and immigrants and this is a fallacy that needs to be corrected. So, the issue of TB in England is now being politically correct—don't blame the immigrants for bringing TB into the country from areas of high TB prevalence.

It seems that some of the British medical authorities (Dr. Zumla and head of the Britain's Protection Agency, Dr. Ibrahim Abubakar) don't realize that the undetected among the immigrant (or visiting) TB patients can become a source of infection not necessarily immediately upon their arrival, but later, after possible activation of their disease or by first infecting the close individuals or members of their families. Denial of the problem due to the political motivations is a disservice to the community, as well as to the social image of the immigrants.

Nearly 40 million non-immigrant visitors arrive in the US annually, but there is no system in place to check these individuals for TB. Unfortunately, this issue was never brought to public attention neither by CDC nor by the media. The solution to this problem first requires its recognition, and then development of a rational and affordable system to check for TB—not only of applicants for immigration to the US (which is in effect now) but also the non-immigrant visitors who come to the US for extended periods. One option can be to place the responsibility of testing for TB on the applicants, requesting that their bacteriological and radiological testing results be submitted with the application, as it is required from those who are applying for immigration to the US.

Major Discoveries, Expectations, and Controversies

Present knowledge of tuberculosis is the result of contributions by many scientists over a long period of time. Some of them were dedicated to their research that cost them in their personal lives, and some of them died from tuberculosis. Scientific publications and the literature written for the general public often address the most important achievement of these great individuals, the real heroes of medicine and science. One can only hope that in the future the names of these heroes will be engraved on the entrance of an international institution for their coordinated efforts to combat TB in the world.

Here is a short list of most important among them:

- René-Théophile-Hyachin Laennec (1781-1826) who invented the stethoscope in 1819
- Heinrich Hermann Robert Koch (1843-1910) who discovered tubercle bacilli in 1882
- Wilhelm Conrad Röntgen (1845-1923) who discovered X-ray in 1895, with subsequent introduction of its use for chest examination and diagnosis of tuberculosis in 1897 by Antoine Béclère (1856-1939)
- Elie Ilyich Metchnikoff (Ilya Mechnikov) (1845-1916) who, in 1882, discovered that tubercle bacilli can harbor and multiply within phagocytic cells
- Albert Calmette and Camille Guérin who introduced the vaccine (BCG) against tuberculosis in 1921
- Selman (Zalman) Abraham Waksman (1888-1973) who discovered streptomycin in 1943.

It was often not a simple task to introduce to the world these and other achievements that represented milestones in the understanding of tuberculosis and in controlling one of the deadliest problems in human history.

These great men were not always seen in a positive light by the scientific community and society, and they often faced serious problems in their personal lives because of their commitment to work. On the other hand, in addition to portraying them as idealistic monuments, some of the reviews also hesitated to address the difficulties they faced because of the reaction to their discoveries by the scientific community and society. The following are a few select stories about the personal lives of some of these individuals, showing that along with being heroes of science, they were just human beings who had to deal with the often unfair way society treated them and their discoveries. These people are now known as founders in the field.

Robert Koch: Tubercle Bacilli As a Cause of Tuberculosis

The infectiousness of tuberculosis was presented by the French military physician, Jean-Antoine Villemin in 1865. He reproduced tuberculosis in rabbits by injecting them with material obtained from TB patients. Robert Koch knew about Villemin's findings but only shortly quoted them seventeen years later in his first presentation about the discovery of tubercle bacilli. Obviously, Villemin's findings encouraged Koch in his research on TB, which he secretly conducted. There were many publications about the life of Robert Koch and his research, beginning with a detailed account in 1910 in *Deutche Medizinische Wochenschrift* by Haffke (#50) up to one of the more recent books by Thomas D. Brock (10).

On March 24, 1882 Robert Koch presented results of his seven-month tightly scheduled research that provided clear evidence that tuberculosis is caused by the tubercle bacilli, *Mycobacterium tuberculosis*. This was not the only discovery made by Robert Koch. He previously discovered the anthrax bacilli, showed the role of staphylococci and streptococci in wound infections, established principles and basic techniques of modern medical microbiology, and later discovered the microbes that cause cholera—at that time called *Vibrio cholerae*.

Among his many achievements as one of the founders of medical microbiology, the most celebrated was discovery of the tubercle bacilli, for which he received many honors from the German government and personally from the emperor. In 1905 he was awarded the Nobel Prize. Not everything was perfect in research by this most celebrated scientist. Among his major failures was the sensational proposal of the *remedy* of tuberculosis, the contents of which was kept secret for a while, but eventually disclosed as tuberculin—the new name for the extract from tubercle bacilli. This *remedy* appeared to be absolutely useless, with unknown and undisclosed possible harmful effect. Only such a giant as Koch could have been forgiven by society for this mistake. Eventually, tuberculin was used for diagnostic skin test purposes only.

In 1882, when Koch decided to present his discovery of tubercle bacilli to the scientific community, he faced a problem—potential opposition from Rudolf Virchow, the famous German pathologist who did not believe that infectious diseases were caused by microbes. At the age of thirty-nine, Koch understood the politics of his society and decided to give his famous presentation at the Berlin Physiological Society meeting instead of the traditional Pathological Society, which was dominated by Virchow.

Ten years later, Koch did not exhibit any political skills when it came to his personal life. After very exhausting days of work, Koch developed a habit of stopping to relax at the nearby Lessing Theater. In 1890 or 1891 he met a young actress (not an artist or an art student, as mentioned by some of Koch's biographers) Hedwig Freiberg, and fell in love with her. The romance between the two began when Koch was forty-seven or forty-eight and Hedwig was seventeen. This affair caused a worldwide scandal in the medical community, a subject of much more attention than the discovery of tubercle bacilli. One of the charges against Koch was that his wife, Emmy Fraatz, played an encouraging role in his career as a microbiologist.

She had assisted him in his laboratory work, and for his twenty-eighth birthday gave him microscope, an extravagant gift at that time. Koch divorced Emmy in 1893 and married Hedwig, but this did not stop the negative gossip in the scientific circles and society. Robert Koch traveled to many places with Hedwig, including the US, and stories from these travels indicated that he was not only a great scientist, but also a sensitive and interesting person. In addition to being a pedantic scientist, Koch had often shown his negative emotional attitude toward his colleagues, especially for those of non-German descent. For example, it is well known that he was particularly negative toward Louis Pasteur.

The complex personality of Robert Koch is addressed in a book by Ilya Metchnikoff (Mechnikov) entitled *Three Founders of Modern Medicine: Lister–Pasteur–Koch* published in Russian in 1915 (Moscow, Nauchnoe Slovo). I have published an English summary of the section of this book related to Robert Koch (11). The title of the book is a good indication of Metchnikoff's respect for Koch. Metchnikoff emphasized that up until that time, all the progress in treatment and control of infectious diseases had been achieved as a result of contributions by Pasteur and Koch. The admiration for Koch in the book was expressed despite unfair, and even disrespectful, treatment Metchnikoff received from Koch.

Ilya Metchnikoff: Tubercle Bacilli As Intracellular Parasites

Elie Metchnikoff (Ilya Mechnikov) was born in Russia in 1845. For political reasons, he emigrated from Russia to Paris, France in 1888, where he spent the last twenty-eight years of his life at the Pasteur Institute, ultimately becoming its deputy director. Paul De Kruif presented Metchnikoff's detailed biography in his famous book, *Microbe Hunters*. There was an interesting detail in description of Metchnikoff's origin. In the English original it said: "Elie Metchnikoff was a Jew and was born in Southern Russia." However, in the Russian translation published during the Soviet era, this phrase was deleted.

In 1882 Metchnikoff discovered a phenomenon called phagocytosis, which is the ability of phagocytes (from Greek "devouring cells") to engulf foreign particles and thus to protect an organism from them. These *wandering cells* included white blood cells. This newly discovered phenomenon was interpreted as a mechanism of protection against bacteria. It was the birth of immunology, but it took many years of hard work and discussions before Metchnikoff's theory of immunity was fully recognized by the scientific community, along with another theory by Paul Ehrlich, who suggested that certain cells of the body produce substances, which today are called antibodies that destroy *the invaders*. In 1908, Metchnikoff and Ehrlich were awarded the Nobel Prize in medicine for their theories of immunity ("cellular" by Metchnikoff and "humoral" by Ehrlich). The history of the discovery of phagocytosis is described in details in my publication, *Centennial of Metchnikoff's Discovery.* (12)

Metchnikoff discovered that tubercle bacilli are not only engulfed by the phagocytic cells, but also able to survive within these cells. Besides the white blood cells, the phagocytic cells also can be found in various tissues; these cells are called macrophages. In the 1970s it was discovered that tubercle bacilli can survive and multiply within macrophages, thus protected from the antibiotics. Bacteria that are able to multiply within the host's cells are called intracellular parasites. Tubercle bacilli can grow and multiply in both types of environment—within the cells and outside the cells in body fluids. Therefore, they are called "facultative intracellular parasites."

Metchnikoff's character could be derived from the style and contents of his book, *Three Founders of Modern Medicine: Lister-Pasteur-Koch*. It was written by a humanist whose feelings about mankind were deeply affected by the onset of WWI. It is interesting to point out that Metchnikoff's admiration for Robert Koch was not affected by the arrogant mistreatment he received from Koch. He just calmly described the event in the following words:

> "Being a leader of a school of young bacteriologists, Koch immediately became an opponent of my theory of immunity to infectious diseases. He gave his students projects whose results could be directed against me.... I went to Koch's laboratory with his senior assistant... The assistant cautiously reported to his boss that I had come by appointment to show him my preparations (showing phagocytosis – LH). "What preparations?" Koch asked angrily. "You better prepare everything I need for today's lecture. I can see that everything is not ready yet". The assistant apologized in a servile manner and pointed at me again. Without shaking hands Koch told me he was very busy and didn't have much time to examine my preparations. I quickly began to demonstrate the slides, which I considered most important.... After a few minutes Koch rose, saying that my preparations did not prove anything and that he did not see any confirmation of my ideas." At the second meeting Koch said: "You know I am not a specialist in microscopic anatomy, I'm

> a hygienist and to me it is not important where the microbes are, inside or outside of the cells". Nineteen years later Koch stated publicly that I had been right at the time I demonstrated my preparations."

Ten years after the meeting in Berlin, the relationship between Koch and Metchnikoff eventually turned into friendship when Metchnikoff hosted Koch and his wife Hedwig in Paris. Koch was already in his early sixties, but did not show any tiredness by attending the theater every evening, which was of special interest to his former actress wife. Metchnikoff invited Koch to the Pasteur Institute where he was welcomed "in the way that kings were honored." The history of the relationship between Koch and Metchnikoff explicitly illustrate the characters of both great scientists. At the same time, these episodes do not fully disclose the character of Metchnikoff.

For many years, I have been intrigued by Metchnikoff's personality and his unusual broad interest in various fields of biology and medicine. I had a collection of his book on subjects such as embryology, biology of old age, philosophy of social life, zoology, nature and prevention of infectious diseases, and immunology. Once, at the request of a Bulgarian Publishing House, in collaboration with two of my colleagues, I wrote and published a book about Metchnikoff. Of course, I could not pass up the opportunity in 1985 to visit the Museum at the Pasteur Institute in Paris, which I knew had an interesting collection of artifacts related to Metchnikoff. The curator of the museum was Ludmila Grabar, a daughter of the famous scientist Pierre (Peter) Grabar.

The museum was dedicated to the memory of Pasteur, and his grave and memorial inside the building is a significant part of the museum. Most of the articles in the museum are related to Pasteur, but some focus on Metchnikoff. Metchnikoff's body was cremated, and the urn with his ashes was placed on the bookcase in the Institutional library, in accordance with in his will ("… where I spent most of my life"). I was very impressed with an interesting drawing of Metchnikoff's profile carved on the window by an unknown artist or student.

Ms. Grabar even took me to where non-exhibited articles were stored. Among them was a bust of Metchnikoff, and Ludmila told me that she did not know who was the artist of this piece. I immediately recognized it as the work of Metchnikoff's wife, Olga, who was a good artist and did pieces of art for her husband. I strongly recommended that this bust should be placed in the exhibit, but I don't know whether my advice was considered.

After the tour, Ludmila asked me whether I would like to meet her father in their apartment near the institute. How could I miss the opportunity and honor to meet the famous Pierre Grabar? It was late afternoon and I had an evening train ticket from Paris to Madrid, but I thought that it would be a short introduction, after which I would be able to catch the train. Pierre Grabar was eighty-seven and retired at the time of my visit. He was so happy to finally have a listener to whom he could speak in Russian and tell a lot of stories from his life in

France. Very soon it became clear that I was going to miss the train, and I had to make a choice: to leave at once and get to the railway station on time, or sacrifice my ticket and stay with Grabar as long as it took. I chose to stay, which later created a lot of problems for my trip to Spain, but I never regretted my choice.

In Russia, Grabar was an officer in the "White Army" fighting the Bolshevics during the civil war. In 1921, he escaped to the west, where he received his education and established a most impressive scientific carrier. He held many important positions and during his time was recognized as one of the founders of modern immunochemistry and immunology. Among his major achievements was the invention and introduction of the immuno-electrophoretic analyses, an important tool in modern research.

Ludmila served tea from the Russian samovar, and the conversation went on endlessly. I was mostly interested in his stories about Mechnikov. Grabar, as a former employee of the Pasteur Institute, knew several of them. One should keep in mind that one of the French traditions of this institution is a very rich folklore, with all kinds of stories and gossip of real or fictional events that took place with many of the employees. Along with all the admiration and respect toward Metchnikoff as a scientist and great humanist, philosopher, and a kind man, Grabar could not resist mentioning that Metchnikoff was also a great womanizer, as he said that he would not miss a skirt.

Referring to the famous picture of Metchnikoff with his two godchildren, officially known as the children of the institutional photographer, Grabar said that everyone knew these children were the biological children of Metchnikoff. Regarding the placement of the urn with Metchnikoff's ashes in the library, Grabar said that such an extraordinary act could only happen because of the request by Metchnikoff's widow Olga, who had a past "special relationship" with Dr. Émile Roux, General Director of the Pasteur Institute.

These and many other stories may not hold any truth, but they may be of interest as a reflection of the social environment in which Metchnikoff lived. At the end of our conversation, I took a picture of Pierre Grabar with a samovar in the background. He was holding a device and said, "This is the very first bacteriological filter made of china, for which I received an award from the Swedish Academy." When I arrived in Denver, I sent the photograph to him, and he wrote on the picture in Russian: "To Dr. Leonid Borisowich Heifets with best wishes, December 6, 1985, Peter Grabar." He sent this photograph back to me. Shortly after I received this photo, Grabar died on January 30, 1986. I was told that I was the last external visitor to visit him at his apartment.

Calmette and Guérin: Vaccine against Tuberculosis (13–15)

In 1900, two French scientists, Leon Charles Albert Calmette, and Jean-Marie Camille Guérin, started their work on developing of the vaccine (later named BCG for Bacilli Calmette-Guérin). The research was based on the idea that the tubercle bacilli (they used *Mycobacterium bovis*) lost their virulence (the capability to cause disease) after cultivation in a broth containing bovine bile. After thirty-nine subsequent cultivation passages on this medium, and eleven years that this work required, many experiments were performed on small animals to confirm the safety of the newly developed bacterial strain.

They vaccinated nine cows with a subsequent infection with a virulent strain. The cows did not develop tuberculosis, which was the basis for the conclusion that the vaccine consisting of live *attenuated* (no longer virulent) strain is safe and can protect from tuberculosis. Unfortunately, at the time of these experiments, the war started in 1914, and German troops occupied Lille where the work was conducted at the Pasteur Institute. The war interrupted the research and had severely affected the personal lives of the two scientists. In 1919 they resumed their experiments, and the hard work continued.

To ensure the safety of the live vaccine they passed their strain through 230 more subsequent broth cultures containing bile, each lasting about three weeks. The safety of the vaccine was evaluated in experiments on various animals, including primates. In 1921 the first newborn child was vaccinated, and in 1924 more than 400 children were vaccinated, and mass production and worldwide use of the vaccine started.

The vaccine was considered fully safe, but in 1930 there was a catastrophe in the city of Lübeck, Germany: sixty-seven children died from tuberculosis and 108 of the 251 subjected to this procedure became ill after being vaccinated. The investigation revealed that there was a tragic mix-up of labeling in the Lübeck laboratory, where a culture of a virulent strain of tubercle bacilli was kept in the same place as the vaccine. The children were given this virulent strain by mistake instead of the vaccine. Obviously, the bio-safety standards known today were not an issue that time. Although the German and French scientists exonerated the BCG vaccine, this episode definitely affected the reputation for the safety of BCG vaccination.

How effective is the BCG vaccine? There was a series of well-organized epidemiological (field) trials conducted mostly in the US and England during the period of 1935-1952, showing variable levels of protection from tuberculosis provided by vaccination. Since these trials, mass production of the vaccine was implemented in many countries. Doubts emerged that variables in handling of it in different countries could have affected the activity of the vaccine strain. To resolve this problem, in 1968 a large field trial was organized in India, and the first reports indicated that the vaccine had no protective efficacy, bur later the results were reinterpreted, indicating that the initial conclusion was mostly due to the inadequate statistical analyses of the result.

The overall statistical analyses assumed that the efficacy of the vaccine was approximately 50 percent protection, which was a two-fold decrease in the probability of contracting tuberculosis among the vaccinated children compared to those who were not vaccinated. The BCG vaccine is used worldwide with more than 100 million doses administered every year. Some countries have a policy of mandatory BCG vaccination, others don't use it at all for mass vaccination (as in the US) for two reasons: one is the uncertainty of its efficacy, and second—because vaccination leads to positive diagnostic skin test which in the past could not be differentiated from results in those who developed the disease.

Presently, there is a different diagnostic procedure available (tasting a blood sample instead of performing a skin test), and BCG vaccination does not interfere with the results of this test. Implementation of BCG vaccination for some groups is being considered. So far, it is a political decision in each country as to whether or not to have a vaccination program. The issue recently became even more complicated because of the concern that as a live vaccine, BCG may not be safe for HIV-infected individuals, and may pose the potential for infection by BCG in individuals with weakened immunity.

Despite the controversy of this issue, the WHO has recommended that in areas with high prevalence of TB, BCG vaccine should be given to infants born to HIV-positive mothers. According to the WHO recommendations, BCG vaccination should be withheld only in cases of symptomatic HIV infection (AIDS). Altogether, in spite of its broad use, the issue of the efficacy and safety of BCG remains quite controversial.

Many scientific groups are making tremendous efforts (including more tremendous cost) in development of new vaccines more effective against tuberculosis than BCG. Even if such experiments are successful, the ultimate answer of the efficacy of a new vaccine will require a clinical (field) trial, and this may be a problem. However, even if successful, introduction of a new vaccine is decades away. Therefore, the hope for effective combat against tuberculosis in the near future cannot depend on such expectations.

Selman Waksman: Antibiotic Era in Treating Tuberculosis

It is well known that penicillin was discovered by accident. Unlike penicillin, the discovery of streptomycin was the result of a targeted search for antibiotic that would kill tubercle bacilli. Moreover, this search was focused on possible production of such an antibiotic by microbes that belong to a group called *Actinomyces*. Some of these microbes are common inhabitants of soil and some can be found in the intestines of animals. The idea of a targeted search came to Waksman's mind in 1932, when a peculiar experiment conducted in his laboratory showed that tubercle bacilli were killed by *something* when they were exposed to soil enriched with manure. (16) Streptomycin was discovered in 1943. However, in the winter of 1941-42 just before its discovery, because of the financial constrains, the budgetary bureaucrats at Rutgers University considered firing Waksman, an "obscure Ukranian-born microbiologist who was getting $4,020 a year for playing around with microbes in the soil". (17)

Selman (Zalman) Abraham Waksman immigrated to the US in 1910 at the age of twenty-two, after realizing that for him as a Jew, higher education was not possible in the Russian Empire. Back in Russia, after taking private lessons, he was allowed to take the gymnasium examination, which provided him with a diploma that opened the doors of the Rutgers College Agricultural in New Brunswick, New Jersey. He received his bachelor of science in 1915, and his master's degree a year later.

At the age of thirty he received his PhD degree from Berkley University on the subject of the biochemical activity of fungi. Back at Rutgers, he focused his research on soil microbiology, particularly on the biology of *Actinomyces*—microbes that by their biological features can be placed between fungi and bacteria. After screening hundreds of strains of *Actinomyces* he found one strain that produced the first, discovered by Waksman, antibiotic called *actinomycin*, which unfortunately appeared to be too toxic to be considered for further development. One of Waksman's important early discoveries was an organism called *Actinomyces griseus*, later reclassified and renamed *Streptomyces griseus*.

Throughout his life, Waksman achieved the status as of one of the guru in general microbiology, attracting dozens of young microbiologists to his laboratory for training and by authoring approximately twenty books and nearly 500 scientific papers. On the background of this success, his major achievement was introduction of streptomycin, the very first anti-tuberculosis antibiotic, which was the starting point of a new era of dealing with the oldest major illness of mankind.

Waksman needed a lot of physical help to screen large numbers of strains of *Actinomyces* in a search for a strain that would produce anti-tuberculosis antibiotic. He had several assistants who did this work, but a dramatic breakthrough appeared in June 1943, when he hired Albert Schatz. This talented twenty-three-year-old recent graduate from Rutgers was the son of a Jewish immigrant from the Russian Empire. He wanted to get a PhD degree in soil microbiology, but was not interested in the search for antibiotics. He did not have a choice if employed in Waksman's laboratory and could only receive his PhD if he found a microbial strain producing an antibiotic active against many bacteria—specifically against tubercle bacilli in experiments directed by Waksman.

Schatz literally worked day and night in a well-organized systematic fashion and applied a very skillful technology for screening thousands of strains. On October 19, four months after he began, he identified two strains of *Actynomyces* from a particular group called *Streptomyces* that showed clear antimicrobial activity! Schatz obtained these two strains from Doris Jones, an employee in another laboratory at Rutgers. She isolated one of these strains from a sick chicken, and another from soil containing manure. Schatz identified both strains as belonging to *Streptomyces griseus*, the species that Waksman had described twenty-eight years earlier. The name of this species became the source for the term *streptomycin*, the name of the new antibiotic. Albert Schatz would receive his PhD!

The first publication on this great discovery appeared in January 1944, with a very modest title, "*Streptomycin, a substance exhibiting antibiotic activity against Gram-positive and Gram-negative bacteria.*" In the title of the report, as is customary among senior American scientists, Waksman placed his name after the names of his two younger colleagues in the following order: Schatz A., Bugie E., Waksman S. (17). The next important step was evaluation of the effectiveness of the drug in treating infected animals. WH Feldman and HV Hinshaw at the Mayo Clinics conducted a large-scale experiment on guinea pigs using streptomycin manufactured by Merck & Co.

After these experiments were completed in January 1945, H.V. Hinshaw and W.H. Feldman performed clinical observations among the first hundred TB patients. (18, 19) These studies and further introduction of streptomycin into practice would not be possible without timely manufacturing of the drug in large amounts in purified concentrated form by Merck & Co. This company had previously established a close relationship with Waksman, which was essential for rapid implementation of streptomycin production. Even George Merck himself was committed to this task, ordering a large number of his employees to be assigned to work with the new antibiotic.

The purified drug supply became available in the US in 1945 and in other countries between 1946-47. The British Medical Research Council conducted a controlled clinical trial and presented indisputable results on the clinical effectiveness of streptomycin. (20) The world received the first miracle drug against tuberculosis! Waksman was invited to give lectures in many countries. As a fourth year medical student I had the honor of attending his lecture in Moscow in July 1946 and to meet Waksman. All who attended the lecture stood in line to shake hands with the famous American scientists. Later, someone made a joke that he would not wash his hand after that handshake. Along with triumph, problems emerged: some of them were related to the drug itself, and others were political.

The political problem arose from the attitude by the coauthor of the discovery, Albert Schatz, toward the glory given to Waksman by the scientific community, as well as society and press, without Waksman giving sufficient credits to Schatz. First, Schatz demanded clarification of his share of royalties from the patent on streptomycin. This issue was resolved in the legal arena in 1950 approving a portion of the royalties (3 percent) going to Schatz personally. In 1952 the Nobel Prize for discovery of anti-tuberculosis treatment was awarded to Waksman for the discovery of streptomycin. This created more negative reactions from Albert Schatz who claimed his rights to be a co-winner of the Prize.

The scientific world was divided in opinions on this issue, and articles and books were written to defend Schatz; the most impressive among them was his own article presented by Inge Auerbacher in a book published after Schatz's death in 2005. (21) Some publications even claimed that the real discoverer was not Waksman but Schatz! Opponents of this view stressed that for many years before Schatz's four-month involvement in the project, Waksman masterminded the whole program and developed the concept that led to the discovery of streptomycin. A storm of letters and media involvement influenced the unprecedented amendment in the decision of the Nobel Committee: Schatz became the co-winner of the Nobel Prize.

Perhaps there were more individuals other than Waksman who deserved the honor of receiving the Nobel Prize for discovery of the cure against tuberculosis. Among them were Drs. Hinshaw and Feldman for their experiments in animals and the first evidence of the effectiveness of streptomycin in TB patients. There was speculation that candidacies of these two scientists were considered by the Nobel Committee, but their names were removed from the list of potential candidates after receiving negative statements from The Mayo Clinic administration, which from the very beginning opposed their involvement in the evaluation of streptomycin.

The reasoning of the Mayo administration is not clear (maybe jealousy), but it was known that many obstacles were leveled against Feldman and Hinshaw to prevent them from work on streptomycin. Their important involvement could have brought a lot of attention to The Mayo Clinic if the administration had appreciated the value of their work for mankind and suppressed some of their narrow-minded personal interests. Perhaps, it is too much to ask from bureaucrats (even doctors) who obtained the executive power to rule over ordinary scientists.

Further Progress in Achieving Cure of Tuberculosis

Another group of potential candidates for the Nobel Prize during Waksman's time was the Swedish scientists led by Jorgen Lehmann and Karl Rosdahl, who developed an anti-TB drug called para-amino-salicylic acid (PAS), a derivative of aspirin. Lehmann proposed the hypothesis of such a drug in March, 1943 in his letter to Ferrosan, a small pharmaceutical company in Sweden. Development of this idea was very slow, not only because of wartime, but because Lehman and his colleagues did not have the involvement of scientists like Hinshaw and Feldman in experiments on animals and clinical research, as well as the close connection Waksman had with such a prominent company as Merck & Co. in the development of streptomycin.

The publication on PAS appeared in January, 1946, much later than the first paper on streptomycin, which was the formal reason for not including Lehman among the winners of the Nobel Prize. In spite of the secrecy under which the activities of the Nobel Committee were conducted, there were speculations that exclusion of Dr. Lehmann was the result of opposition by one of the members of the committee simply motivated by academic rivalry and jealousy, as described by Frank Ryan. (23)

More important than the political controversies around the Nobel Prize, were the real problems from observations on the extensive use of streptomycin around the world. One of the problems was the toxic effect of the drug. It caused deafness in some patients, particularly in those who received streptomycin for extended periods or in too large doses.

Another problem was that in a substantial number of patients who did not recover within a short period of time under treatment with streptomycin, the tubercle bacilli would become resistant to streptomycin, and the drug became useless for these patients. Eventually, it was evident that emergence of resistance to any anti-tuberculosis drug is inevitable if the patients are treated with only one drug. This discovery later led to the need for simultaneous use of several anti-tuberculosis drugs.

At the same time when streptomycin and PAS were introduced for practical use, the third anti-tuberculosis drug, isoniazid, emerged. In January 1952, three pharmaceutical companies (Bayer, Squibb, and Hoffman-La Roche) simultaneously presented this new anti-TB drug, indicating that it was more effective than PAS and streptomycin. In 1950 Isoniazid was developed as a derivative from a previously discovered drug named Conteben, or Tibone, or TB-1, which belonged to a large group of chemical compounds called thiosemicarbazones. Tibone was synthesized in Germany by a group of chemists at Bayer led by Gerald Domagh (1895-1964). Domagh was a recognized expert in the field of drug discovery. In 1939 he received the

Nobel Prize for discovery of the sulfonamide Prontizil which was effective against streptococcal infections.

Studies in the 1950s by the three companies mentioned above indicated that isoniazid appeared to be much more active and less toxic than Tibone. The situation was on the edge of a large lawsuit for the patent among the three companies who claimed priority of the discovery of isoniazid. Suddenly, all three companies found that in fact they were not the first to synthesize isoniazid but two chemists, Hans Meyer and Josef Mally, in 1912! This powerful drug was just sitting on the laboratory shelves and waiting for more than thirty years for its rediscovery.

Discovery of the original invention resolved the controversy about the patent rights (which none of the companies received). Isoniazid started its worldwide march as an important component of anti-tuberculosis treatment and is now being manufactured by all three companies. Introduction of isoniazid also resolved the problem of drug resistance to any agent (including isoniazid) emerging after single-drug therapy with either of the drugs. In the early 1960s based on an application of the three-drug combination, a new approach was developed for the most effective therapy of tuberculosis (streptomycin+PAS+isoniazid).

Over the years more anti-TB drugs were discovered, and the most important among them were pyrazinamide (1952), ethambutol (1963), and rifampin (1966). It is important to stress that introduction and proper use of all these drugs would not be possible without their evaluation in clinical trials. British Medical Research

Council (MRC) under the leadership of Drs. D'Arcy Hart, Wallace Fox, and Denis Mitchison conducted most of this work. MRC developed a methodology of the so-called "controlled clinical trials" to achieve the most objective results, and organized such trials in East Africa, India, Hong Kong, and Singapore.

Series of trials were conducted during the period of more than half-a-century to address the major questions regarding proper implementation of the anti-TB drugs. This fundamental research provided unquestionable proof of true efficacy of the evaluated drugs. Among the findings is evidence that three or four drugs should be used simultaneously during the first two to three months of therapy in a new patient to avoid development of drug-resistance of his bacteria. Justification of the six-month treatment regimen (instead of the twelve-month regimen previously used) by incorporating rifampin and pyrazinamide in the treatment schedule was one of the most important results of the MRC clinical trials.

It became the basis of the current recommendations for the so-called short-course standard treatment regimen that consists of two months of the intensive phase of treatment with four drugs (rifampin, isoniazid, pyrazinamide, and ethambutol or streptomycin) followed by four months of treatment with rifampin and isoniazid. One must remember that this standard regimen is intended for new patients whose bacteria are susceptible to the administered drugs. It is important to stress, that methodology developed by the MRC is currently used by various research groups for evaluation of new drugs and improved treatment regimens. The principle of combined therapy introduced by the MRC remained a key principle of tuberculosis therapy today, although different drugs can be included in various combinations.

History of Tuberculosis, Lessons to Learn (22-25)

Contagious illnesses were known in ancient times and were addressed in the Bible. The focus was only on the very obvious, such as skin lesions on people who were often labeled as lepers; many of them perhaps may not have had leprosy but various fungal skin infections. The plagues of smallpox, diphtheria, typhus, enteric infections, black plague, cholera, and leprosy during the Middle Ages and current epidemics of influenza and HIV/AIDS have made significant marks in the history of mankind.

From ancient times, tuberculosis has affected humans. This is confirmed by examination of some of the four thousand year old Egyptian and Peruvian mummies. For example, approximately six percent of Peruvian mummies have shown signs of tuberculosis. Some authors speculated that during the period of intensive cattle breeding activities, particularly in ancient Egypt, *Mycobacterium tuberculosis*, the organism that causes tuberculosis in humans, evolved from *Mycobacterium bovis*, a related species causing tuberculosis in cattle.

Recent genetic studies overruled this theory, showing that *M. tuberculosis* is a more ancient species than *M. bovis*, and it is more likely that *M. bovis* evolved from *M. tuberculosis.* (26) A review of recent discoveries regarding the origin of TB suggests that this infection may have affected the human race for the last nine thousand years, and may have originated in pre-historic times between two and three million years ago (27) Very often the ancient mummies excavated in Middle East area had bone and joint lesions, typical for tuberculosis. This finding is an indication that tuberculosis may have often been in the form of disseminated infection affecting many organs throughout the body.

Perhaps, often in ancient times death could not be correctly identified as associated with a specific illness. This is especially true of tuberculosis because of the variable characteristics of this disease and of the broad range of its clinical manifestations. Until the twentieth century and up to the recent significant progress in this field, diagnosis of tuberculosis has not been a simple task.

During ancient times and the Middle Ages, tuberculosis was not recognized as a major health problem affecting any of the major historic events or social life. Tuberculosis was not recognized as influencing political life, although, as mentioned by Chretien, the history of Europe could have taken a different path if such personalities as King Louis XIII of France, Richelieu, or children of Catherine de Médici, and other important royalties and politicians had not died from tuberculosis.

The role of tuberculosis in social life in Western Europe changed with the development of a new environment in the seventeenth and eighteenth centuries, a situation that was not common during the previous history of mankind. Growth of overcrowded cities combined with extreme poverty, ignorance of basic hygiene, and possible contagiousness of many illnesses provided favorable conditions for the spread of infectious disease.

During the period of more than 200 years, particularly in eighteenth and nineteenth centuries, the epidemic of tuberculosis grew and spread throughout Western Europe, with a peak in 1800 and the first half of the nineteenth century. The TB epidemic accounted for the deaths of approximately 25 percent of the Western Europe population and was labeled as the White Plague. (22)

Among the factors that contributed to the spread of tuberculosis in Europe in the seventeenth through the nineteenth centuries was the fact that the contagious character of this illness was not clearly recognized until Koch's discovery of *Mycobacterium tuberculosis* in 1882. Death from tuberculosis, which was frequently confused with death from other illnesses, was often associated with some hereditary or behavioral conditions. Many authors described tuberculosis as a wasting disease or consumption, sometimes without clear distinction from other such illnesses.

It is amazing that for a long time, even after the sensational reports by Robert Koch, ignorance regarding the infectious character of tuberculosis dominated not only the public's general knowledge but also the medical community. One example of a rather anecdotal view was *Medical Adviser* by R.V. Pierce, a book written to educate the public, published in 1891, nine years after the discovery of tubercle bacilli! The list of possible causes of tuberculosis in this book is very long, and included:

> spermatorrhea, dyspepsia, nasal catarrh, colds, suppressed menstruation, bronchitis, syphilis, retrosession of cutaneous affections, measles, scarlatina, malaria, whooping-cough, small-pox, …masturbation, excessive venery…insufficient diet…dampness, prolonged lactation…fast life in fashionable society…

There was no mention of tubercle bacilli.

Scrofula, a form of tuberculosis affecting neck glands, along with more severe generalized and lung forms of the disease, was widely spread during the period of the White Plague. Perhaps, in many patients it could have been the manifestation of generalized tuberculosis. Since swollen glands were visible, the diagnosis of *scrofula* was apparent. Throughout the centuries, a myth circulated in Europe that this illness could be cured by the touch of royalty, and thousands of pilgrims travelled to England and France to be touched by the monarch.

This practice peaked in the seventeenth century and ended at the beginning of eighteenth century—never reaching the shores of America. The power of royalty to cure *scrofula* was considered the result of anointing and coming from God. Of course, it could not be expected from an elected president of the country. So far, none of the US presidents have claimed acting on the behalf of God. Otherwise, let the imagination flow if the ritual of touch would come to America.

In the nineteenth century, the tragic outcome of tuberculosis, most often called *consumption*, inspired some poets and composers to create such characters as Violet in Verdi's *La Traviata* and Mimi in Puccini's *La Bohème*. It is interesting to note, that *La Traviata*, the novel by Alexandre Dumas *La dame aux Camélias* (which title some critics interpreted as *The Fallen Woman*) and the opera by Verdi were created in the 1850s, long before the cause of tuberculosis was discovered and before the knowledge became available that it was an infectious disease.

Nevertheless, the original description by Dumas and in most of the performances, the manifestations of the illness of Violet in the first act and the death in the third act are depicted the distinct appearance of a generalized form of tuberculosis. Puccini's opera was staged in 1896, long after the discovery of tubercle bacilli, but it was influenced by a libretto written in 1848 after the 1830 autobiographical collection of stories, *Scenes de la Vie de Bohème* by Henri Murger. Through most of the opera Mimi's illness was portrayed with all the symptoms of pulmonary tuberculosis (also called *consumption*) with coughing and suffering, and accompanied by very dramatic passages of the music. The thin, pale faces of both heroines were considered beautiful, and the lyrics of both operas emphasize this beauty.

Another piece of art, which was also influenced by Murger's stories, is an 1858 photograph by the famous French photographer Felix (Gaspar-Felix-Thaumahon) Nadar. The photo is of a woman sitting in a chair, partially wrapped in fabric. This photograph is preserved in the Metropolitan Museum of Art (Met), and was labeled by Jacques Chretien in his book (25) as "Mimi". There are speculations by the experts at the Met, that Murger's girlfriend Lucille (who died from tuberculosis) served as the model for this famous photograph. One way or another, there is a traditional association of this photograph with Murger's stories, hence, with TB.

In the literary classic, *The Magic Mountain* (1924), which was written much later but long before the cure against tuberculosis was discovered, Thomas Mann was inspired by his impressions of the social environment of the Davos sanatorium in the Swiss Alps and the individual stories from the tuberculosis patients there. This famous book was sometimes called "The Epic of Disease". It reflected society's perception of tuberculosis as another Romantic's illness, and that those afflicted with tuberculosis were considered sensitive, brooding, and creative individuals. The book contains very broad speculations and deep philosophical thoughts about such topics as the meaning of life, health, illness, death, sexuality, morality, and the duality of European civilization. The book was awarded the Nobel Prize in literature in 1929.

Historically, romanticizing some illnesses was not new. In the past, tuberculosis was the subject of this approach, along with the widespread perception in the 19th century that it affected highly intellectual individuals. This view was enhanced by the fact that many celebrities died from tuberculosis, including John Keats, Nicolo Paganini, Robert Louis Stevenson, the entire Bronte family, Johann Wolfgang von Goethe, Frederic Chopin, Béla Bartóc, Percy Bysshe Shelley, Ralph Waldo Emerson, Robert Burns, Henry David Thoreau, Carl Maria von Weber, Elisabeth Barrett Browning, Baruch de Spinoza, Edgar Allan Poe, George Orwell, Amadeo Modigliany, Franz Kafka, Igor Stravinsky, Fyodor Dostoyevsky, and Anton Chekhov. One can only imagine how much the world missed because of the premature death of these individuals.

Death from tuberculosis of many well-known personalities may have affected not only the development of culture, but also some historical occurrences as well. For example, the course of Russian history may have taken a different path if the heir to the Russian throne George had not died in 1899 in Nice from tuberculosis, which he contracted during his travels through the southern Europe.

The tuberculosis epidemic eventually spread from Europe to major American cities, and in the 1880s severely affected the Native Americans, particularly when they were confined to reservations and forced to live in barracks and small fixed huts, and having intensive contacts with the White settlers, many of whom brought TB from Europe to America. In the mid-1800s, tuberculosis accounted for 24 percent of deaths in Providence, 23 percent in New York, and 15 percent in Philadelphia. Death rates among Native Americans accounted for approximately nine percent of their tribal populations in 1886. (28)

An innovative idea, introduced in 1854 by Hermann Brehmer, was that tuberculosis could be cured by rest and exposure to fresh air. Thus, sanatoriums were established in Switzerland, Italy and other countries. In the US the proposal of sanatoriums was developed by Edward Livingston Trudeau (1848-1915), an idea to isolate TB patients to prevent the spread of the disease and to provide appropriate treatment. The first famous sanatorium in the US was the Adirondacks Cottage Sanatorium established in 1885 at Saranac Lake, New York. Based on his personal experience as a surprising survivor of TB, Dr. Trudeau developed a program that included a healthy diet and outdoor exercise. This Sanatorium grew to a small village at the turn of the century, providing affordable home and free medical service to poor individuals.

About 650 sanatoriums (hosting more than 600,000 patients) were in existence in the US in 1923. Among them, the sanatorium in Arkansas, open from 1910 through 1940, was among the most efficient. Not all sanatoriums had such a reputation, and some of them were viewed as just a place where patients were dumped to die. In the early 1960s the idea of sanatoriums began to fade away because of availability of effective anti-tuberculosis drugs and hopes that a cure could be achieved without prolonged and expensive isolation and hospitalization.

Eventually, it was shown that under treatment with anti-tuberculosis drugs, a dramatic decrease in the number of bacteria excreted by the patient could be achieved within weeks and even days. Switching to ambulatory treatment instead of hospitalization created a problem of patients' no-compliance (non-adherence) to the prescribed treatment regimen. Many patients started feeling better and stopped taking the prescribed medications long before completion of therapy intended for a period of many months. That was the main reason (besides the problem of availability of drugs in some communities) that introduction of highly effective anti-tuberculosis medications did not result in significant changes in the prevalence of tuberculosis.

Massive non-compliance with the prescribed treatment led to the emergence and spread of epidemics of drug-resistant tuberculosis. It was too late and too unpopular to go back to the principle of the sanatoria, where patients' compliance with the prescribed treatment could have been easily observed. Eventually this problem was addressed by the introduction of the directly observed therapy (DOT) to be applied for a period of six months of treatment. Despite the positive effect of this approach, the worldwide outcome of the current TB control system was limited and far from desirable. The general decline in the TB prevalence was minimal and the growing spread of drug-resistant tuberculosis continued.

Perhaps, closure of the sanatoria in the past was premature, and the unpopular long held idea of re-establishing the TB sanatoria is currently gaining new interest. The recently published review on this subject has a remarkable title, *The Global Rise of Extensively Resistant Tuberculosis: Is the Time to Bring Back Sanatoria Now Overdue?* (29)

There is a definite need to develop a new system to treat MDR and XDR cases, and sanatoria would be a good place to guaranty good compliance of patients with the described treatment, and, most importantly, to implement the individualized therapy with antibiotics to which the bacteria in these patients are still susceptible. This idea can be realized if there are laboratories capable to determine the drug-susceptibility pattern of tubercle bacilli from these patients. One can anticipate opposition to such suggestion, mostly for political reason, since it would contradict the WHO strategy and the principle of the standard treatment regimen, unless it is labeled as an extension of the DOTS program.

Even after introduction of the anti-tuberculosis antibiotics, tuberculosis in the US remained a serious health problem and no one was completely safe. First Lady, Anna Eleanor Roosevelt died from tuberculosis in 1962. How could that happen? Was it a medical mistake? In 1999, the Institute of Medicine issued a report that about 98,000 patients die each year from medical mistakes, which makes it the fourth leading cause of death in the US, and it is possible that one such victim was Mrs. Roosevelt. Her medical record was sealed from 1965 until 1990, and the review of her story revealed the difficulties that physicians at Columbia-Presbyterian Hospital, one of the best American institutions, had in its history an incorrect diagnosis of tuberculosis in this high profile patient (30).

For a long period of time (since The First Lady was diagnosed with *aplastic anemia* and later with a "fever of unexplained origin," (or FUO) she was treated with prednisone which may have weakened her immunity. Two months before her death, suspicion arose that she may have had *miliary tuberculosis*, a disease in which the tubercle bacilli spread throughout the body due to the weakened immunity. This diagnosis was neither confirmed by X-ray examination, nor laboratory testing. However, as a precaution, she was treated (although not very systematically) with two anti-tuberculosis drugs, isoniazid and streptomycin.

On autopsy the final diagnosis was "*disseminated miliary tuberculosis*," and it was stated that, according to the literature of that time, *miliary tuberculosis* was correctly diagnosed before death in only 25 percent of cases. The final note in this tragedy is that tubercle bacilli, isolated from Roosevelt's bone marrow, appeared to be resistant to both isoniazid and streptomycin, and treatment with these drugs would not have helped even if applied in a timely manner.

The tuberculosis history in the US would not be complete without addressing the events that took place in Colorado at the end of nineteenth century. Denver's dry climate and high altitude attracted people seeking relief from all kinds of illnesses, including tuberculosis. Denver became known as the *Mecca for Consumptives*.

New arrivals, mostly poor people, crowded the city and often died in the streets without being able to receive any medical help or general assistance. The city became a place of growing prevalence of tuberculosis. Most of the business activities in Denver flourished by serving the needs of the miners bringing gold and silver in exchange for various services provided to them.

The public and newspaper attention was more focused on stories related to cowboys, gunmen, and outlaw adventures, competition among the six famous bordellos and other events in the "Red Light District". Others focused on the tragic events related to the silver crisis, such as the crash of Mr. Tabor's enterprise in 1893, or the personal romantic story of Baby Doe Tabor, the adventures of Doc Holliday, and other famous personalities. The problems with large numbers of TB patients arriving to Denver did not appear to be the primary focus of that society.

In the background of public indifference to a devastating public health problem in 1880s and 1890s, the Denver Jewish Community perceived the situation of TB patients dying in the streets as intolerable and initiated activities that led to the establishment of the National Jewish Hospital. Along with a substantial number of members of the community were two individuals, Ms. Frances Wisebart Jacobs, and Rabbi William S. Friedman, who deserve special tribute for initiating these activities. One of Ms. Jacobs' concerns was the problem of indigent patients suffering from tuberculosis and the need for a place for them to be treated. Unfortunately, Mrs. Jacobs died in 1892, before her dreams of having a TB hospital in Denver were realized. A man of action, Rabbi Friedman, promoted the idea that concern for the sick and indigent had always been an element of Jewish tradition.

The funds were collected within the Denver Jewish Community and other cities, and the first hospital building was constructed in 1893. Unfortunately, due to the financial problems caused by the "silver crisis" of 1893 the hospital could not open until six years after its construction. Finally, in 1899 thanks to the Jewish charitable organization "B'nai B'rith" (Sons of Covenant), the hospital began admitting TB patients. This organization provided financial support for at least 50 years, and also organized fund raising in many Jewish communities and organizations around the country. Rabbi Friedman was one of the first presidents of National Jewish and served for fifteen years until his death in 1944.

National Jewish became a unique hospital in the US that provided free admission to indigent TB patients for nearly fifty years. From the very beginning, National Jewish was proclaimed as a non-sectarian organization. Subsequently, the hospital has received financial support not only from Jewish groups and communities, but also from a large number of Christian and secular organizations, as well as private donors. Through the years, the hospital has undergone several name changes, including the most recent in July 2008, *National Jewish Health*. The word Jewish has remained in the each name change as a tribute to the role of the Jewish Community in starting this institution and continuing financial support, although only a small number of employees or patients were, or are, Jewish.

The history of the early years of confronting tuberculosis in Denver is addressed in detail by Dr. Jeanne Abrams in her book entitled "*Blazing the Tuberculosis Trail*" (31) . According to this monograph, three more institutions (sanatoria) addressing the problem of tuberculosis in Colorado were subsequently opened. They were: the Jewish Consumptives' Relief Society (JCRS) in 1904, Evangelical Lutheran Sanatorium in 1905, and the Swedish National Sanatorium in 1908. Another large TB sanatorium in Colorado was the Modern Woodmen Tuberculosis Sanatorium in Colorado Springs, which provided free treatment to thousands of patients between 1909 and 1947.

In 1889 the National Tuberculosis Association in the US formed a committee called The National Association for the Prevention of Tuberculosis (NAPT) with the goal of educating the public on the real nature of tuberculosis. As a result of World War I, tuberculosis epidemics were devastating in Europe. This provided the impulse in 1920 for establishment of the International Union Against Tuberculosis as a leading international institution in understanding the optimal ways to deal with the problem. Aside from the support of the network of sanatorium activities, there was not much these organizations could implement, until the anti-tuberculosis drugs were discovered. At the end of the 19th century, the idea of reporting TB cases was brought to light with an initiative by Dr. Herman

Biggs of New York City, but the national case reporting system was not established in the US until 1953.

In 1959 the National Tuberculosis Association organized the famous Arden House Conference (in Harriman, New York), a meeting of eighteen top American experts. The Conference had ambitiously planned to eliminate tuberculosis in the US, and among the primary recommendations, was emphasis on the widespread application of the anti-microbial therapy (chemotherapy) as a public health measure. The concept of directly observed therapy to guarantee patients' compliance with the prescribed therapy was not in the air yet, and ideas of proper laboratory developments for rapid diagnosis and drug susceptibility testing were still in the embryonic phase.

The subsequent events that occurred over the years did not support the optimistic expectations of the Arden House Conference. At the time of the Arden House Conference, about 65,000 new cases of tuberculosis were reported annually in the US. The number of new cases declined to approximately 50,000 annually in the 1960s, followed by a long period of fluctuation. The decline in the prevalence of TB in the US was slower than anticipated due to the unexpected changing situation, including the emerging problems of dual TB+HIV infection epidemic and spread of drug resistant tuberculosis.

Critical analyses of the Arden House Conference recommendations presented by the authors from CDC in view of the subsequent events over the years may be of interest to understand the changes in perception of the evolving situation by the leading medical professionals (32). Contrary to previous perceptions, the authors of this review have reached the conclusion that tuberculosis elimination in the United States will not be feasible until both technological advances and social justice allow control systems to be applied throughout the world.

The history of tuberculosis since the 1970s, in the background of advanced knowledge of the biology of tubercle bacilli and the discovery of a growing number of anti-tuberculosis drugs, was predominantly the history of politically motivated decisions by various organizations, committees, and governments. For example, in the Soviet Union, any statistics on tuberculosis was considered a State Secret, because the prevalence of TB in the country was very high, contrary to the idea that tuberculosis is a social system-related illness and should not have been a problem under socialism but was only supposed to have high prevalence in a capitalistic society.

Another feature typical of a totalitarian system was that in the Soviet Union (and now in Russia) it was mandatory that any proposals for control measures, selection of drugs to treat TB, procedures (even details of the lab tests), and general policies must be approved and implemented by the Ministry of Health. This was a reflection of the traditional Soviet attitude of mistrust of the medical professionals in their ability to think and make their own decisions.

In the US, any proposal on treatment, laboratory testing, etc. from the CDC or any other specialized committee is only a recommendation. Nevertheless, the nature of human beings often dominate the mind of the American as well as other medical professional, no different from the one in Russia, with the attitude of anticipation that the proper authority would "approve" any procedure or standard treatment regimen, which eliminate the necessity to think, make decisions, and take responsibility.

Historically, tuberculosis has been one of the most neglected world health problems. Although proper analyses of the situation in developing countries was not available for many years, some reviewers suggested that this neglect was motivated by the substantial decline in the number of tuberculosis cases in industrialized countries. In 1990, the World Health Organization (WHO) and its European branch organized a symposium entitled *The Last Fight Against Tuberculosis Until Elimination*. It was an indication that outside of industrialized countries the need for programs to control and not eliminate tuberculosis was not in the view of the world health leadership.

The attitude began to change in 1993 after the WHO declared tuberculosis a global emergency. Statistical data on the actual spread of tuberculosis in the world were based on various estimates rather than on verified data and took into account the number of new cases of TB emerging in the world annually. According to the review by F. Dobrinewsky, A. Pablos-Mendes, and M.C. Raviglione (33-34), the average global rate of new TB cases (incidence) in 1995 was estimated to be nearly 152.0 per 100,000 of the surveyed population, and mortality of 51.6 per 100,000. Since then, these indicators have been fluctuating, depending mostly on the populations selected for the surveys.

Since the 1950s, tuberculosis epidemics no longer represent a natural process. Anti-tuberculosis drugs were developed, and TB became a curable disease. It is proper to say that the situation when no treatment was available was bad, but inadequate and incomplete treatment in many countries today is even worse. A new type of tuberculosis emerged; drug-resistant TB, and eventually, multidrug-resistant TB (MDR-TB). In addition to drug-resistance, two more important elements have changed the face of TB: one is the fact of TB and HIV merging pandemics, another is extensive travel of people around the world.

An alarming situation occurred in the US in the late 1980s. There were seven outbreaks of MDR-TB in Florida and New York City—approximately 200 cases, mostly in hospitals and correctional facilities, with a mortality rate of 72 to 89 percent! Most of the patients were co-infected with HIV, and the results of laboratory testing indicated that the bacteria were resistant to the drugs used for treatment, but arrived too late, often after the patients' death. Dramatic measures, with a very high cost, have been implemented to stop these epidemics and to prevent then from occurring in the future. Was this a lesson to prevent TB outbreaks in the future? A report by the *Hoffpost Miami* published on July 11, 2012, indicated that there is a major TB outbreak in Jacksonville, Florida. This outbreak has already resulted in thirteen deaths among the more than 100 TB patients, but mostly among the homeless.

Importance of the laboratory testing for timely detection of patients having MDR-TB was not recognized in 1980s at either national or international level. The opinions about the importance of the emerging situation of drug-resistant TB in the world medical community in 1990s were far from consensus, even after the first objective information about the extent of the problem of MDR-TB was presented in 1998 as a result of a survey in 35 countries (33, 34). One of the WHO publications (35) suggested that it has still not been documented that primary MDR contributes significantly to the treatment failure rate of WHO standard regimens. Subsequently, such evidence was presented in a number of studies indicating that the substantial prevalence of primary drug resistance decreases the overall cure rate of the standard treatment regimen (36-38).

Often different authors expressed opposite opinions based on the same statistical data of the first survey. Some of the authors used a world median of 1.4 percent rate of primary (in new patients) MDR-TB cases as an indication of the low importance of the MDR problem, while others stressed that MDR at that time already emerged in 104 countries, the rates of primary MDR were above 8 percent in 24 of 35 surveyed countries, and above 24 percent in eight of them.

According to the 2010 WHO Global Report (WHO/HTM/TB/2010.3), an estimated 440,000 cases of MDR-TB emerged globally (with 150,000 deaths) in 2008, almost 50 percent of them in China and India. About six percent of MDR was diagnosed among new cases in twelve countries, and 50 percent or more among the previously treated cases in five of these countries. Eight countries reported XDR-TB in more than 10 percent of MDR-TB cases. Despite the optimistic reports by WHO and some countries, the situation in the world is getting worse with the emerging epidemics of drug-resistant tuberculosis in many parts of the world.

What Do We Know About Tuberculosis Today?

Our current knowledge about tuberculosis is based on many discoveries made over a period of more than 100 years, and the history of only a few of these major discoveries were presented above.

For thousands of years, tuberculosis was considered a hereditary disease, and until the 19th century, many physicians could not accept the fact that it was a contagious infection. Today there is no longer doubt that tuberculosis is an infectious disease caused by bacteria commonly known as tubercle bacilli. In fact, it is a group of bacterial species named *Mycobacterium tuberculosis* complex. Within this group four species may cause tuberculosis in humans (*M. tuberculosis, M. bovis, M. africanum, M. canettii*), but can also cause tuberculosis in cattle, cats, and some other animals. The most common cause of disease in humans is *M. tuberculosis*.

Few other mycobacterial species (*M. microti, M. caprae, M. pinnipedii)* are found to be the cause of a similar disease in animals, but they most likely cannot cause disease in humans. The most usual clinical manifestation of tuberculosis is lung disease, but it can also affect other organs and can appear as a generalized infection when the bacteria are spread throughout the body through the bloodstream. It is well established now that individuals who are diagnosed with active tuberculosis (when the lungs are involved) are contagious, and the TB infection can be transmitted to others, particularly in a closed environment, by small droplets of sputum generated by coughing, sneezing, laughing, etc. Consumption of products from animals (such as milk, cheese, or meat) having tuberculosis is another way of contracting the disease.

There is a large group (approximately 80 species) other than tubercle bacilli mycobacteria that exists in the environment (water, soil) called non-tuberculous mycobacteria (NTM) that can be found in clinical specimens from humans. Some of them can cause disease, including lung disease. Individuals with a normal level of immunity rarely develop an illness caused by these bacteria. On the other hand, those that have certain pre-disposing conditions are vulnerable to infection with these environmental bacteria. Among these pre-disposing conditions are chronic bronchitis and other chronic lung diseases, history of heavy smoking, diabetes, and AIDS. Unlike tuberculosis, patients with NTM are not infectious and NTM are not transmitted from person to person.

How contagious is tuberculosis? It is known that even under conditions in a close environment, not all individuals that have been in contact with a TB patient necessarily become infected. Perhaps, only about 40 percent of them, depending on the period of exposure and the level of immunity, may be a reflection of the individual's genetic make-up. Only a small proportion (approximately 10 percent) among those infected with tubercle bacilli that have a "normal" level of immunity will ever develop an illness, or active tuberculosis—most of them not immediately, but throughout their lifetime.

Until such event occurs, and for nearly 90 percent of those infected who would never develop active disease, the tubercle bacilli may lie in dormant in the body without causing any symptoms. This is called "latent tuberculosis," and these individuals are not contagious and cannot transmit the infection to others, unless the dormant tubercle bacilli are activated (in the above mentioned 10 percent cases). Nearly one-third of the global population (about two billion people) has latent tuberculosis, but its prevalence in some countries is much higher than average, thus, in case of activation, represents a potential reservoir of TB infection in the community.

The situation is different in cases when the immunity is not "normal" but affected by various factors, such as malnutrition, diabetes, many other chronic illnesses, but most of all by HIV infection. In individuals that are HIV-positive (even before any symptoms of AIDS can be detected) an infection with tubercle bacilli most likely would rapidly progress into active tuberculosis.

In individuals that have already had the latent form of tuberculosis, infection with HIV could activate the dormant tubercle bacilli in their body, which would transform the latent form of the disease into active tuberculosis. The potential risk of this occurrence is very high, close to ten percent annually. Therefore, the current worldwide epidemic of HIV/AIDS has changed the whole situation with tuberculosis, including an overall increase in the prevalence of new cases from new infection and due to reactivation of TB in individuals with the latent tuberculosis.

Since the 1940s and up to the present time, at least twelve antibiotics to treat tuberculosis have been discovered, and so far the disease is considered almost 100 percent curable if the patient has tubercle bacilli susceptible to the administered drugs and if the patient is in compliance with the prescribed treatment regimen. Treatment period for a new case usually requires administration of three or four drugs for a period of two-three months, followed by administration of two drugs for a period of four-six more months.

The total treatment period lasts at least six months, if bacteria are susceptible to the administered drugs. Patients' adherence even to this simplest treatment regimen became a problem, not fully recognized in time by the medical community. This non-compliance often resulted in development of resistance of the patients' bacteria to some or all administered drugs, and a new phenomenon emerged—epidemics of drug-resistant TB.

Population of tubercle bacilli in a patient, even before any therapy with an antibiotic, is very diverse. It always contains very tiny proportions of natural mutants resistant to various antibiotics. Treatment of a patient with an antibiotic eliminates the vast majority of the bacterial population, but the small sub-populations of the pre-existing natural mutants resistant to the administered drug may survive. As a result of this selection, a drug-resistant strain would multiply to replace the previous drug-susceptible bacteria. To prevent this occurrence, for the purpose of affecting bacterial sub-populations resistant to various drugs, modern treatment of tuberculosis patients is based on administering three or four drugs at the same time.

Another important standard is to administer these drugs for a sufficient period of time, because an insufficient period of treatment (or the drugs' dosing) may not completely eliminate even the drug-susceptible bacteria. As a result, the patient may have a mixed population consisting of susceptible and drug-resistant bacteria. In the situation, when drug-resistance develops as a result of inadequate treatment, it is called *primary drug-resistance*. Another scenario is when drug-resistance is a result of infection from a patient who already has drug-resistant bacteria: this is known as *secondary drug-resistance*.

The history of tuberculosis presented in the previous chapter demonstrated that the magnitude of the tuberculosis epidemics and their potential effect on social life in the past and up to the present time was largely underestimated by society. According to the WHO estimations, there is more TB today than at any other time in the history of mankind, with 2 billion people infected with tubercle bacilli. In 2007, approximately 1.7 million deaths from TB worldwide were reported, but it is estimated that in reality the annual number could have been close to 2 million. More statistical data regarding the tuberculosis situation in the world is listed in Appendix 3.

Emergence of MDR and XDR is a new phenomenon that occurred during the past two decades. MDR-TB is defined as multi drug-resistant TB when bacteria are resistant to at least the two most important drugs, rifampin (RMP) and isoniazid (INH). XDR-TB is defined as extensively drug-resistant TB, when in addition to RMP and INH the bacteria are also resistant to any of the quinolones (such as ofloxacin, levofloxacin, or moxifloxacin) and to at least to one of the injectable second-line drugs (amikacin, kanamycin, capreomycin).

Patients harboring drug-resistant bacteria became a source of infection to others, and an epidemic of a difficult to treat disease is spreading around the world. This alarming situation requires additional measures, both administrative (such as treatment according to the Directly Observed Treatment standards to ensure the patients' compliance with the prescribed treatment regimen), and development of laboratory services to detect, in a timely manner, patients with drug-resistant

TB for proper timely treatment and prevention of the spread of drug-resistant tubercle bacilli.

Emergence of HIV/AIDS epidemics in the 1980s dramatically changed the whole picture, because HIV affected the immunity, making the HIV-infected individuals extremely vulnerable to tuberculosis at a very early phase of the HIV infection, before any clinical symptoms of AIDS can be detected. The most frequent scenario, especially in developing countries, is that many of those who had latent TB infection and most likely would never develop active TB, had suddenly converted into active TB cases due to the immune system being weakened by the HIV infection. Also, in cases of exposure to TB, the HIV-infected individual most likely would develop active tuberculosis instead of the most usual (without HIV) dormant (latent) TB infection. In some areas, such as sub-Saharan Africa, at least one-third of all new cases of TB were recently attributed to the HIV epidemic.

Part 2:

With a Glance into the Future

Recycling of the White Plague

The sign in front of me read: "You are not welcome."

The post-surgical boot on my leg said: "Please, seat this man!"

However, the waiter standing in front of me said, "I'm sorry, we don't have room for you."

I had arrived at Antwerp shortly after having surgery on a ruptured tendon—a consequence of my mountaineering adventures. The welcome was most unkind. The weather was rainy, my foot was aching, my stomach was rumbling, and this man would not allow me sit in what appeared to be an almost empty hotel restaurant. I complained to the management pointing to my inability to go out in the rain and that after all, I was a guest. Finally, I was served, but the attitude made for a bad first impression. As I continued my stay in Antwerp, indeed, the city seemed to say, "Go away."

Why did I even go there, with all these sufferings, to this inhospitable place called Antwerp?

The motivation for this trip was my ambition: I was invited to give a keynote lecture at an International Colloquium, and could not miss an opportunity to receive this honor and to express my professional views at this prestigious gathering. Among the attendees were representatives of the WHO, International Union Against Tuberculosis, and leading TB experts from many countries around the world.

The International Colloquium was entitled, "Tuberculosis, The Real Millennium Bug," and was organized by the Institute of Tropical Medicine in Antwerp on December 14-17, 1999. It was something new—one of the first international gatherings to recognize the emerging problem of drug-resistant tuberculosis. At the Plenary Session of this colloquium, I delivered a keynote lecture (The Henri Taelman Lecture) that was titled, "Recycling of the White Plague: Prescription for Disaster".

It was provocative in both its title and its contents. Taking advantage of this high-profile colloquium, one of the first international gatherings recognizing the emerging problem of drug-resistant tuberculosis, I would be criticizing the DOTS strategy introduced by the WHO five years earlier, explaining its inadequacy for the growing prevalence of drug-resistant TB.

The abstract of my lecture was included into the Program Book of the Colloquium, but the full text of the lecture did not appear (contrary to initial intention) in the subsequent publication *Multidrug-resistant*

Tuberculosis edited by the organizers of the Colloquium, my good friends Drs. Ivan Bastian and Françoise Portaels (39). Most likely, this deletion was motivated by political reasons, since the lecture contained too much criticism of the WHO strategy.

Ten years have passed and several of my critical statements were proven to be correct. Although a number of significant improvements in the WHO's recent policies, at least in words, were made regarding the WHO strategy to control TB, the actual situation in the world still remains troublesome. Today, even more so than ten years ago, the epidemics of drug-resistance are posing a threat of growing prevalence of incurable tuberculosis in some areas of the world. The current control measures appeared to be insufficient to prevent such a development, and a warning about a new white plague still seems timely. That is why I borrowed the title of this chapter from my lecture presented ten years ago.

Six years before the Colloquium in Antwerp, in 1993, the World Health Organization (WHO) declared tuberculosis a global emergency. Unfortunately, for a long period of time, this declaration did not receive needed support from the world governments. In 1994 the WHO launched the "Framework for Effective TB Control (WHO/TB/94.179)", which became known as "WHO TB Strategy," and is currently known as, "Directly Observed Therapy, Short-course" (DOTS). The initial response by the leadership of many countries was far from enthusiastic.

To address the concern of the cost, the WHO leadership promoted the idea that the DOTS strategy was fully affordable, even in countries with limited financial resources. This strategy was further enforced by a number of additional documents issued by the WHO. One of them was the new Stop TB strategy issued in 2006 as "The Global Plan to Stop TB, 2006-2015". This document stressed as a success of the program the fact that 36 million patients have been treated under DOTS-based services since 1995.

But how many millions of TB patients have not been treated, either with or without the DOTS strategy? M.A. Espinal and M.C. Raviglione from the WHO in their most recent review indicated that the DOTS-based programs successfully treated 49 million TB patients between 1995 and 2009 (40). These authors also addressed the evolution of the WHO strategy from the original DOTS to the enhanced DOTS program, and now, to the Stop TB Strategy. This evolution was needed in response to the constantly emerging challenges. For example, "DOTS was not designed to properly address the threats of HIV and multi-drug resistant TB (MDR-TB)."

The five major elements of the *original* DOTS strategy introduced in 1995 included:

1. political and financial commitment of the government to the established National TB Program
2. uninterrupted drug supply with appropriate management system

3. standardized monitoring and evaluation system of the patients
4. treatment under directly supervised administration of drugs to all newly diagnosed patients, using the standard combination of drugs ("short-course")
5. direct microscopic smear examination of the patient's sputum for the presence of tubercle bacilli as a basic criterion for the TB diagnosis and as an indicator of recovery when the smear becomes negative.

The primary concept of the original DOTS strategy was to ensure compliance with the prescribed treatment by directly observing patients taking the medications. There were no arguments against this primary principle, but some of the other elements of this strategy produced controversies and inevitable arguments, which led to modification of formulations of some of these elements over the years.

Introduction of the DOTS strategy occurred in the background of uncontrolled worldwide broadening application of anti-tuberculosis drugs, which resulted in the inevitable emergence of drug-resistance of tubercle bacilli in many patients. For many years, the importance of this problem—in particular the role of patients with primary (initial) drug resistance as a source of drug resistant tuberculosis infection—has been underestimated. Therefore, drug susceptibility testing of the patients' isolates (particularly in new patients) was not considered a priority measure in TB control.

Statements from leading national and international organizations illustrated this neglect. For example, the American Thoracic Society (ATS) and Centers for Diseases Control and Prevention (CDC) published the following joint statement, "Given the low prevalence of drug-resistant *Mycobacterium tuberculosis* in most part of the United States, the cost of routine testing of all initial isolates is difficult to justify" (41). Severe outbreaks of drug-resistant tuberculosis in the US in the late 1980s and early 1990s changed this attitude, and testing of initial isolates for drug susceptibility became mandatory (42). For many years, this lesson did not influence the attitude outside the US. Moreover, with introduction of the DOTS strategy in 1994-95, new arguments emerged against the worldwide use of drug-susceptibility testing. One argument was that many countries could not afford the laboratory arrangement needed for such testing. Another reason was that according to the original DOTS strategy, the focus was on using smear microscopy as the main diagnostic tool to detect most infectious patients. It did not matter that this testing was only able to detect less than 50 percent of the culture-positive patients (even less in HIV-infected patients), but culture isolation and drug-susceptibility testing were not considered for broad implementation.

In 1997, the WHO Guidelines for the management of drug-resistant tuberculosis contained the following statements, "Susceptibility testing is not recommended in all new cases of smear-positive pulmonary tuberculosis…since it is not practical, it is expensive, and it is useless" and "The level of resistance…is lower in primary than in acquired resistance. This is why primary resistance hardly affects the outcome of treatment with a WHO standard regimen…"

Misguided statements, based on the intention of promoting the idea of the primary role of microscopic smear examination over culture isolation and drug susceptibility testing can be found in some of the WHO publications. For example, a document entitled "Guidelines for the Management of Drug-Resistant Tuberculosis" was published in English and in Russian (43).

A footnote on page seven of the English version states: "Occasionally, with single-drug treatment or inappropriate drug combinations, resistance can occur after only two or three weeks. It may be necessary to consider this when prescribing drug combinations for an individual patient." The text of the same footnote in the Russian edition states: "Exclusively rare, the poly-resistance is being detected in new patients, e.g., in patients that have never been treated before and have been infected with poly-resistant M. tb."

"In the majority of countries, new cases caused by such poly-resistant bacteria represent a very insignificant proportion of all new TB cases with primary resistance." This so-called translation from English into Russian was, at best, inaccurate. It is obvious that the intention of this misrepresentation was to convince the Russians to overcome their critical views of the DOTS strategy (particularly toward microscopy as the only diagnostic tool, as they perceive this program) and to subscribe to this WHO policy.

A tendency to present unjustified optimistic views can be damaging for timely introduction of updated policy changes. For example, some authors referring to the report of the first worldwide 1994-97 surveillance on prevalence of drug-resistance dismissed the importance of this phenomenon, based on the finding that the frequency of primary MDR calculated as a median for thirty-two countries was only 1.4 percent, which justified no changes in the WHO policies and no actions to address the problem. Different statistics could have been derived even from the same survey: the overall rate of primary resistance of all types was above 8 percent in twenty-four of thirty-five surveyed countries, and above 24 percent in eight of them.

The rates of primary MDR were already high in seven countries (from 4-6 percent to 14.4 percent). Predictably, the rates of drug resistance since then were increasing in many countries. Underestimation of the problem was not universal at that time, and there were diverse opinions with regard to understanding of the need to broaden attempts for detecting patients harboring drug-resistant tubercle bacilli.

In 1999, the leading WHO expert Dr. Mario Raviglione stated in an interview to the *NY Times* (October 29, 1999): "In our zeal to implement DOTS everywhere, there was no clear policy in the program to take care of multidrug-resistant TB. Now we realize that something more must be done." The journalist called this statement "an unusual endorsement from

WHO's leading specialists." Despite this admission, it took ten years until policy changes were introduced in the recent 2010 WHO document. And still no clear plans for implementation of a new approach!

The initial WHO recommendation focused on the microscopic smear examination of the sputum as the simplest and the least expensive method to detect the most contagious patients that expectorate in their sputum a large content of tubercle bacilli, detectable even under the microscope (more than 1,000 bacteria per ml of sputum). The recommendation at that time reflected the predominant opinion that patients who produced smear-negative sputum did not play a significant role as a potential source of TB infection. This view appeared to be false.

Special observation conducted in San Francisco discovered that such patients did infect others even if they were treated in a timely manner. It is not known how much more important they are as a source of infection to others in countries where they are not diagnosed as having TB because of negative microscopy smear results and therefore are not treated. One should keep in mind that many TB patients expectorate up to 20.0 ml and more of sputum every day. Not infectious, if the sputum contains less than 1,000 bacilli per ml? Culture isolation and drug susceptibility testing of the patients' bacteria was not a part of the original WHO recommendations intended for developing countries, thus having about half of all new patients undetected and unattended.

Due to criticism from many developing countries, the WHO finally modified its recommendations by recognizing that the microscopic smear examination has limited value. The importance of modern bacteriological methods is now fully recognized, including culture isolation for complete detection of all tuberculosis patients in the community, and especially for timely detection of patients with drug-resistant tuberculosis.

It appeared that the obstacle to development of modern laboratories was not insufficient funding, but rather the local and international bureaucratic attempts to create universal rules and to be credited for such development, along with unreasonable and sometimes corrupted distribution of funds. In all industrialized countries, culture isolation and determination of drug susceptibility/resistance of the tubercle bacilli isolate is a standard element of health care. Eventually, the problem came to light that WHO recommendations were not the same between industrialized and developing countries.

Laboratory diagnosis is now elevated (at least in statements) by the WHO to the most important element of the DOTS strategy and expressed as "case detection through quality-assured bacteriology", instead of just microscopy as it was in the past. It now stresses that culture and drug-susceptibility testing should be introduced in a phased manner (44). Unfortunately, so far there are no actual plans to implement these good intentions. Moreover, the new WHO documents contain a number of controversial statements and recommendations that don't fit into the declared new approach toward the role of bacteriology. In the 2011 review from the above-mentioned WHO perspective, Espinal and Raviglione emphasize the situation with patients diagnosed by smear-microscopy. In other words, they ignore the other 50 percent of patients with negative smears.

In this review, the smear-positive patients are often listed as *infectious patients* implying the outdated view (without directly saying) that the smear-negative patients are *not infectious.* This article stresses that in order to prevent outbreaks of MDR-TB, "approximately 70% of prevalent *infectious* [emphasis added] patients should be detected and treated." Again, under *infectious* the authors meant those who are smear-positive. So far, no one has proved that the smear-negative patients are not infectious, but the opposite.

Another example of insufficient transformation of the WHO strategy is that the latest WHO document quoted above still suggests decentralization of diagnostic services along with a recommendation that each country should have a Reference Laboratory. This formulation is inherited from the past documents when decentralization meant multiple microscopy stations, and the function of the Reference Laboratory was defined as a focus on supervision and quality assurance of operation of these stations.

Still, the wording of the new policy does not address the idea of the most effective comprehensive testing under the direct submission of raw specimens to large properly equipped laboratories, not just literally Reference Laboratories. Complete case detection (and detection of patients having drug-resistant bacteria) through quality assured bacteriology cannot be achieved without appropriate modernization of the laboratory services when all new patients (not only those with positive microscopy results) are subjected to culture isolation and timely assessment of drug-susceptibility of their bacteria. This is possible only through having large properly equipped laboratories with submission of the patients' specimens directly to such laboratories. So far, such a plan has not been expressed in the WHO documents.

As mentioned above, one of the important elements of the original DOTS strategy was to treat *all* newly diagnosed tuberculosis patients with a standard treatment regimen (under direct supervision). This regimen consisted of a combination of three or four drugs (rifampin, isoniazid, pyrazinamide, and ethambutol) during the first two-to-three months (intensive phase of therapy) followed by treatment with only two drugs (rifampin and isoniazid) for four to six months. If properly implemented, this standard treatment regimen should provide a cure for more than 90 percent of patients that have bacteria fully susceptible to all drugs incorporated into this regimen.

Unfortunately, this regimen was recommended indiscriminately for all patients, not taking into account the likelihood that some of them may already have tubercle bacilli strains resistant to the administered drugs. This type of resistance could have been a result of improper documentation of previous unsuccessful treatment or because the person was infected from a TB patient that had drug-resistant bacteria—a phenomenon called primary or initial drug-resistance. Apparently, the WHO managers either underestimated this fact, or just did not express any concerns about this problem.

Contrary to initial expectations, DOTS strategy did not prevent the growing intensity of drug-resistance among patients who had undetected initial resistance to some of the administered drugs. The argument was that proper implementation of the DOTS strategy, particularly implementation of the standard treatment regimen for all patients, was supposed to prevent the spread of drug resistance, and even make it virtually impossible for a patient to develop MDR-TB (35).

A group of authors referring to their experience in Peru stated, "It is not true that DOTS makes it virtually impossible to cause a patient to develop MDR-TB" (45). They demonstrated how patients with initial resistance only to RMP or INH developed additional resistance to other drugs through DOTS treatment—a phenomenon they labeled as "amplified effect of short-course therapy." Escalation of this phenomenon into the MDR epidemics became unavoidable through blindfolded (without drug susceptibility testing) universal application of the standard regimen.

As a result, new epidemics emerged: multi-drug resistant (MDR), and most recently, extensively drug-resistant (XDR) tuberculosis. These epidemics could have been prevented if all new TB patients were tested for drug-resistant bacteria and if they were treated not with the standard WHO combination of drugs, but subjected to an alternative treatment regimen based on the individual drug susceptibility pattern of bacteria recovered from each patient. Such individualization is opposite of the standard regimen, and it was condemned by the WHO administration.

Therefore, by initiative of Dr. Arata Kochi (at the WHO), scientists from Harvard University (Dr. Farmer's group) suggested the same approach under the pretense of the politically correct name: DOTS-plus Strategy. In fact, it was based on the DOT principle, but it was not DOTS at all, because it did not suggest a standard regimen for all patients, but individualization based on drug susceptibility test results in each patient. There were no objections from the WHO, but neither was there any significant efforts made to implement it, mostly because of the cost.

The core of the new STOP TB Strategy launched by the WHO for 2006-2015 was DOTS, and the recent WHO reports stressed the successful implementation of this program. As mentioned above, one of the indicators of this success was the fact that between 1995 and 2006 about 36 million (now 49 million) have been treated under DOTS-based services. Again, no reference is given to the number of TB patients that were not treated at all. Major points of this new strategy included expansion and enhancement of high-quality DOTS, and addressing the problems related to the TB+ HIV and MDR-TB epidemics. The plan has established targets to be achieved by the year 2015, one of which is to "halt and begin to reverse the incidence of TB by 2015". One of the indicators of successful implementation of this plan quoted in the recent WHO reports is that In 2008, an estimated 62 percent of new smear-positive cases were treated under DOTS – just short of the 70-percent target. In other words, at least 50 percent of all new patients (the smear-negative cases) were not detected and not treated. Therefore, one can estimate that in 2008 only about 30 percent of all new TB patients were treated. Can this level of "success" lead to a significant decline of TB in the world? Can any success in prevention of epidemics of drug-resistant tuberculosis be achieved without testing the new patients for initial drug resistance? Can any success be achieved by ignoring the needs of TB detection in smear-negative patients as a potential source of infection?

Regardless of new or modified policies and despite the celebrated progress based on certain "indicators" mentioned above, it seems that the epidemics of drug resistant tuberculosis are growing, and emergence of incurable TB in some areas of the world is becoming a reality. Perhaps, the overall prevalence rates of TB in the world will start declining after 2015. Perhaps, more patients will be treated under the DOTS guidelines. Perhaps, one can anticipate further increase in a proportion of patients with smear-positive sputum specimens treated under DOTS standards, which is one of the indicators of the success of the DOTS strategy. At the same time, the number of patients harboring drug-resistant bacteria will continue to grow, up to 1.6 million cases annually by the year 2015, as predicted by the WHO report of 2010.

Someone said that plagues are like taxes,they are inevitable, but the public's attention with regard to the emerging diseases is concentrated only on exotic new infections. A very entertaining and detailed book by Laurie Garrett, *The Coming Plagues* (1994), gives a description of many new emerging infections, including a dramatic story about Ebola infection. At the same time, this book tells very little about MDR-TB, except the brilliant phrase: "The emergence of novel strains of multidrug-resistant TB came amidst a host of changes, whistles, and bells that should have served as ample warning to humanity. But the warning fell on unhearing ears". Maybe the warning was not loud enough? And that is, despite a popular quotation that MDR-TB is like *Ebola With Wings* (46). Like Ebola, if untreated MDR-TB is fatal, but unlike Ebola, it is spread through the air, and it is already killing more people than Ebola.

The most prominent among the TB experts, Dr. Lee B. Reichman in collaboration with journalist Janice Hopkins Tanne published in 2002 a book entitled, *Timebomb: The Global Epidemic of Multi-Drug-Resistant Tuberculosis*. The warning of the danger of the emerging epidemics of drug-resistant TB was very loud this time, much louder than the previous warnings and despite the fact that even the term *Timebomb* in this connection was earlier introduced by Dr. Michael Iseman, but perhaps not as loud as this time. The authors of the book also skillfully borrowed the above-mentioned term "*Ebola With Wings*" as the title for the first chapter of the book.

For many years, Dr. Reichman has been the most vocal expert in the field, warning of the coming danger of the drug resistant TB epidemics. He was among the very first experts to call attention to the merging epidemics of TB and AIDS and to the need of combining efforts against both. Even in the 1970s, when TB was considered a problem of the past, Reichman spoke about the possible epidemics of TB in the US. As early as 1971, he testified before a Congressional Committee, stressing that TB was not just a problem of the past, but also a threat to the future. Unfortunately, the issue was not elevated at that time to a public health priority. Efforts by Reichman and others for advocating the need for the highest level of attention to TB as an international problem are well summarized in his book.

Dr. Reichman is also the most adamant proponent of the DOTS Strategy, and the book's attention is focused on the needs for vigorous implementation of this WHO strategy (in its original version described above) as a key element in preventing the epidemics of drug-resistant tuberculosis. Implementation of the Directly Observed Therapy in Newark, New Jersey, through extreme efforts by a team of the outreach workers is described in detail in a special chapter.

Particularly impressive is the description of the genuinely heroic efforts by Ms. Rebecca Stevens in reaching "difficult" patients around the city for implementation of the Directly Observed Therapy. The program was highly effective, with up to 96 percent cure rate. The chapter is titled, "DOTS in the real world," but the problem is that Newark is actually not the "real world" if one keeps in mind the situation in developing countries where DOTS was targeted.

Also, Newark's strategic model of dealing with TB is really not DOTS as defined in the WHO documents. The original DOTS strategy was intended for low-income countries, but the sputum specimens in New Jersey from all TB patients were tested not only by smear examination but also by culture isolation and drug-susceptibility testing in two high quality laboratories—the Institute and/or at the State Laboratory. If drug-resistance was detected in some patients, they were not treated with the standard regimen but with an individualized combination of drugs selected on the basis of drug-susceptibility testing. Therefore, the Newark model could have been called DOT, but not DOTS.

Although the important role of proper laboratory activities in prevention of epidemics of drug-resistant TB is now fully recognized by the WHO leadership, there are still debates going on regarding whether to have full scale laboratories in the developing countries. New development in the field of rapid TB diagnosis and detection of drug resistance is often targeted to support the idea of possible de-centralization of the laboratory services, hence, not to depend on full scale laboratories (such as in New Jersey) in developing countries with limited resources.

An example of such development is the invention of an automated system (GeneXpert MTB/RIF test) developed by the Cepheid Company. The main point of this development is that the new system provides an opportunity to perform the test at the doctor's office, thereby providing results within two hours, without any laboratory involvement. The testing provides information for most of the sputum specimens by reporting whether the sputum contains tubercle bacilli and whether the bacilli are rifampin-resistant, which is considered a marker for MDR. The opportunities provided by this procedure sound very attractive, but there are too many problems, as addressed in the chapter, "Hopes in India," using the situation in India as an example, and in more detail in the chapter, "Laboratories—The Ultimate Weapon."

India has the capability to establish a system of full-scale TB laboratories for complete testing—including all reasonable microbiological and molecular methods—of specimens submitted to them directly from the patients. Such laboratories would not only provide high quality results within the shortest possible turnaround time, but would also be much more cost efficient than the current system of microscopy stations or introduction of the Cepheid system in every doctor's office. So far, one of the obstacles of such development is a tendency towards political correctness by agreeing with some of the WHO recommendations for de-centralized laboratory services.

The attitude toward establishing full-scale TB laboratories in other high TB burden countries is either equal to that in India or even worse. It seems that there is no hope that the epidemics of MDR and XDR will gain enough attention and proper management without changing the existing philosophy and without elevating the standards in this field to the level that already exist in the industrialized countries.

What is the probability that the recycling of the old TB into incurable disease will continue? The pessimistic point of view is that it will continue until it reaches dramatic proportions. You may call MDR-TB "*Ebola With Wings*," but in the eyes of the majority, it will still be known as TB. Society will not recognize the real danger of the coming new white plague as long as this incurable disease does not personally affect those who influence the public and governments' perception.

Until then, the process of recycling of the *old* TB into the incurable TB epidemic will continue. Therefore, the efforts of the world scientific community should concentrate on global education concerning the coming danger. Huge funds are needed to prevent the new epidemic, and these funds will not be allocated until after the new epidemic hits the world economy and life. As I stated above, in my presentation (1999) cited above, there were no signs that the attitude toward the new threats of a pandemic of incurable TB were changing at that time, even among the leading medical professionals. Unfortunately, it is not much different now.

African Tragedy

Walking through the rain forest was no fun. The skies were cloudy, and although it was only twenty-eight degrees Celsius, the extreme humidity physically dominated me. The condensation on the tree leaves constantly dripped, creating a noisy shower. I was called to visit a patient on the outskirts of a village in the *Ituri* forest. Reaching the destination did not give me any relief; the temperature in the hut was stifling and the putrid odor of the patient's perspiration permeated the air.

I saw a man lying on an elevated mat, his body wasting away. I estimated him to be in his thirties. He was shivering and his thin face was wet with perspiration. From time to time he coughed, spitting out bloody sputum, and what appeared to be pieces of his lung. I carefully placed my stethoscope on his chest. The sounds I heard indicated there were numerous cavities in his lungs. He was semi-conscious and because his condition was beyond help he would soon die from tuberculosis. That was one of the few cases of tuberculosis that I observed in more than twenty villages of *Ituri* forest during my expedition to the former Belgian Congo in 1962.

Severe health problems other than TB and HIV were the focus at that time. I was there as a member of a medical delegation from the Soviet Union, and as a young physician, I faced the challenge of handling patients with a variety of illnesses unknown to me. Often the situation was quite dramatic, especially in cases when the cure was not available. Once when driving with my team through one of the villages, the locals stopped us and demanded that we tend to a patient.

A young woman was sitting on the threshold of her house with her arms lifted up, screaming and crying. She suffered from extreme pain in her forearms and could not tolerate any touch to her skin. The cause of her agony was a neurological manifestation of leprosy, a widely spread illness at the time in the Congo. I could not do much, but the local people expected some magic. Fortunately, I had some painkillers, and gave her a dose before continuing on my trip. There were much more dramatic situations to come.

At the time tuberculosis was not a major problem. Most of the cases were among children, and all were extremely severe. The diagnosis was not difficult to establish; merely a physical examination and microscopic smear examination of sputum were sufficient. Most of these patients were dying from tuberculosis, and the sight of an emaciated patient, such as the one previously described, left an indelible lifetime memory. Statistical data fade in the wake of such memories.

Many years later, in 1994 and 1995 after moving to the United States, I visited Africa again. I observed a completely different situation than in the 1960s, there were not just a few cases of tuberculosis, but TB epidemics along with HIV/AIDS epidemics.

Health problems in Africa have a long and painful history. Devastating epidemics of malaria and high prevalence of parasitic illnesses, leprosy, sleeping sickness, skin infections, combined with insufficient supply and quality of food and constant wars between tribes resulted in a substantial decline in the African population at the beginning of the twentieth century, followed by significant population growth during the subsequent period of almost a hundred years.

Tuberculosis was not prevalent in the sub-Saharan African countries and some areas of North Africa before 1860 (47). After many years of the colonial period, TB cases were rare among the inhabitants of small remote villages, unless they were exposed to the infection through contact with Europeans. The increasing spread of TB in South Africa only began after 1908, along with the increasing number of Europeans moving to sub-Saharan Africa.

At that time and during the subsequent decades, tuberculosis appeared to be one of the most neglected world health problems. Some reviewers suggest this neglect was motivated by a substantial decline in the number of TB cases in industrialized countries, while proper analyses of the situation in African and other developing countries was not available for many years. It became clear in mid-1980s that the emergence of the HIV/AIDS epidemic would lead to the most dangerous health problem of dual TB+HIV epidemic, affecting both industrialized and developing countries.

In 1994-95 the WHO declared a strategy known as DOTS, which is described in the previous chapter. Despite the growing financial and logistic support from the international community, response by the leadership of many African countries to this strategy was not timely enough. Partially, it was due to lack of understanding of the magnitude of the problem, but more so because of preoccupation with the political struggle and military conflicts. In addition to the overwhelming corruption in several African countries was concern for the cost. To at least overcome this problem, the WHO leadership promoted the idea that the DOTS Strategy was fully affordable even in countries with very low income. Over a few years, officials from most of the African countries accepted, at least formally, the proposed WHO strategy.

In 2005 the WHO Regional Committee for Africa comprised of forty-six member states declared TB an emergency in Africa. The declaration stated that the number of new TB cases in most African countries quadrupled since 1990 and continued to rise. It stated that although at that time Africa had only 11 percent of the world's population, it accounted for more than a quarter of the global burden, which was estimated at 2.4 million TB cases and 540,000 TB deaths annually.

The Declaration called for more commitment by the member states to the DOTS program, although it stressed that implementation of this program depended on external financial support, particularly from the Global Fund to Fight AIDS, TB, and Malaria (GFATM).

Some statistical data (based on estimations by mathematical modeling) that illustrate the burden of TB in Africa are presented in the Appendix 3. As it is stated in the WHO report, the lack of actual information on the spread of drug resistance in Africa is a result of inadequate laboratory capacity to perform diagnostic testing among TB patients.

Some of the original WHO recommendations appeared to be inapplicable in Africa. One of them stated that treatment of TB patients should be done in an ambulatory setting without hospitalization. It was unrealistic for some of the patients in rural areas to go to the ambulatory facility to receive supervised treatment. The mandated exception was to allow these patients to be treated in hospitals. On the other hand, many patients were reluctant to be hospitalized because of the stigma associated with the fear that their families and neighbors would think that they had AIDS—the commonly known cause for hospitalization in Africa.

Application and reasoning for some other standards of the WHO strategy became the subject of controversy and criticism during recent years with the background of emerging epidemics of multi-drug-resistant TB (MDR-TB), and most recently—extensively drug-resistant TB (XDR-TB). The overall consensus is that contrary to the initial expectations, DOTS strategy did not prevent these epidemics.

The opinion expressed at the 2007 World Lung Conference was that current efforts to control drug-resistant TB epidemics were failing. Some experts felt that this failure was morally reprehensible and that drug-resistant TB was a man-made phenomenon (S. Lewis and P. Farmer). At the same time, there are not many specifics addressing the initial cause of the MDR epidemics. It is still not politically correct to question some elements of the DOTS strategy as a possible cause of these epidemics.

South Africa was the first country where an outbreak of TB, caused by so-called extensively drug resistant tubercle bacilli (XDR-TB), was reported in 2007 (48). These XDR bacteria evolved from MDR because of inadequate management of patients with MDR. Outbreaks of the XDR epidemics may signal the emergence of incurable (with available antibiotics) tuberculosis.

Because of extreme involvement of politics combined with the flow of money from other countries and international groups, the decision making process often falls into the hands of people who don't have enough expertise in TB but are ambitious in taking credit for any introduced measures. Sometimes, this attitude can reach an epidemic level.

Acronyms, such as MDR and XDR, are very popular these days. Perhaps, another acronym can be suggested for the problem of incompetent individuals in the leadership often dominating the fight against

TB. I would suggest labeling it XAI, which stands for *"extensive arrogance combined with ignorance"*.

An important element of the original DOTS five-item strategy is that TB diagnosis should be based primarily on microscopic examination of the sputum smears, because it is simple and inexpensive, which makes it attractive to low-income countries. The major problem with this approach is that use of microscopy as the only diagnostic tool excludes any possibility of knowing whether the newly diagnosed patients have drug-resistant strains of tubercle bacilli. That is in addition to the fact that the best quality microscopic examination fails to detect TB in more than 50 percent of TB patients.

The alternative is that in addition to microscopy, to implement culture isolation of tubercle bacilli from sputum. This would require the availability of laboratory services and associated substantial cost, which exceeds the cost of a smear examination. Detection of drug resistance/susceptibility pattern of the patient's bacteria is impossible without having culture of tubercle bacilli isolated from the sputum. In all industrialized countries culture isolation and determination of drug susceptibility/resistance of the isolated tubercle bacilli is a standard element of health care. Eventually, the problems of inconsistent recommendations for industrialized and developing countries were exposed.

Under criticism from many developing countries, the WHO finally modified its recommendations by recognizing that microscopic smear examination has limited value. The importance of modern bacteriological methods is now fully recognized, including culture isolation for complete detection of all TB patients in the community, and especially for timely detection of patients with drug-resistant TB.

It is refreshing to learn that in a most recent interview (49) Dr. Mario Raviglione, director of the STOP TB department of the WHO, stated, "We felt that laboratories are the weak link in TB control and particularly MDR. Without laboratories we cannot make the diagnosis of MDR." He also stated that there is now a program in place to increase the diagnostic capabilities in 27 developing countries.

The problem now is how to achieve this goal. The obstacle is not only insufficient funding; the US and other countries contributed large sums. In addition, some countries have enough of their own resources that are just not focused on TB control. The problem is driven by attempts of local and international bureaucracy to create universal rules and to be credited for such development, along with unreasonable and sometimes corrupt distribution of funds. Tuberculosis has always been a political problem, and it is not surprising that even now, political issues dominate this major health problem rather than rational decision-making.

In my previous publications, as well as in many of my presentations, I relentlessly emphasized that the key element in preventing and diminishing the drug resistant TB epidemics is to have proper laboratory services that would be the least expensive element of the TB control program. The reason for this point of view is that only proper bacteriological examination of all new TB patients would provide detection of individuals who carry drug-resistant bacteria.

If the lab results can be available within a short period of time, such testing would ensure timely adjustment to the initial standard treatment regimen and make more efficient treatment of patients with drug-resistant bacteria. This system would help alleviate the spread of drug resistant strains of tubercle bacilli. One of the obstacles to this approach is the tendency to have a network of small laboratories (close to the patients) or, as this approach is labeled, to have a decentralized laboratory system with many microscopy stations or so-called *seeding stations*.

Under these conditions, none of the small laboratories could afford any modern equipment or even proper bio-safety protection. I have tried (unsuccessfully) to convince a number of my colleagues that only a centralized system with direct delivery of sputum specimens from patients to well equipped laboratories with highly qualified personnel would resolve the problem of obtaining results within the shortest possible time. This system would guarantee high quality testing, and would be much less costly than a de-centralized system. It is not uncommon for even the best laboratories in many countries to not have proper bio-safety standards, and in some places the laboratories have become the source of infection for laboratory workers. There is a need to create model TB laboratories to demonstrate their cost-efficiency and productivity, but also as educational facilities for TB microbiologists.

The situation has become even more dramatic with the development of the devastating epidemic of Acquired Immunodeficiency Syndrome (AIDS), which appeared to be the most significant factor in triggering the growth of tuberculosis prevalence in African countries. Infection with the Human Immunodeficiency Virus (HIV), that causes AIDS, affects the immune system in such a way that an individual becomes highly vulnerable to tuberculosis, either by activating a dormant TB infection or causing an individual to become sensitive to a new infection with tubercle bacilli.

Tubercle bacilli can survive in the body system for many years without causing any clinical symptoms. This is called latent tuberculosis infection (LTBI). Millions of people (perhaps, two billion, which is one-third of the world population) have LTBI and represent a potential reservoir of TB if the tubercle bacilli are activated. HIV infection is now the major factor that can transform LTBI into active tuberculosis. Long before any symptoms of AIDS can be detected, development of active TB may be the first clinical manifestation that the person is infected with HIV. In people who did not have LTBI but have HIV, an infection with tubercle bacilli will most likely result in active tuberculosis rather than in the LTBI status. As a result, an intensive epidemic of HIV infection in African countries became the major cause of the rise of the tuberculosis prevalence. Tuberculosis became the primary cause of death among patients with HIV/AIDS.

The AIDS epidemic not only became a medical problem, but also a political one, even more so than that of tuberculosis. Over the years, politics surrounded such issues as the history of AIDS, its nature as an infectious disease, and measures for prevention and treatment. It was concluded that HIV causes AIDS. It should be mentioned though, that few scientists, including Drs. Peter Duesberg and David Rasnick, and some African political leaders (for example, former President of South Africa Mr. Mbeki) denied (even in 2000) the role of HIV as a cause of AIDS. This view contributed to the delay in implementation of appropriate prevention and treatment measures. A scientist at the University of Cape Town (Nicoli Nattrass) blamed Mbekii's administration policy as the cause of more than 300,000 deaths in South Africa.

There are other theories that also diverted attention from the real problems. One of them is the so-called *conspiracy theory*, suggesting that HIV was intentionally spread to diminish the black population in Africa and in the US. Another theory suggests that the AIDS epidemic in Africa is a result of colonialism.

It is generally accepted that HIV originated in Africa, most likely an infection from chimpanzees and monkeys that often carry the so-called Simian Immunodeficiency Virus (SIV), which may have evolved into HIV either in these animals or in humans infected with SIV. It is estimated that such an event may have occurred in 1930s or even much earlier. The first confirmed AIDS cases in Congo were traced back to 1959 and 1960 by examining the preserved blood and tissue samples; it has been estimated that by the1960s nearly 2,000 people had been infected with HIV. The HIV/AIDS epidemic in Africa reached a noticeable epidemic in the early 1980s. Since then, more than 15 million people have died from AIDS, and more than 22 million in Africa are now infected with HIV.

In the US, the beginning of the AIDS epidemic was first recognized in 1981 as a strange illness among a small number of gay men, and an average of two new cases every day was reported in 1982. The term AIDS was introduced and the problem brought to the public's attention. It is not clear how the HIV infection was brought to the US. Some scientists suggest that it came via Haiti, but others argue that HIV infection was brought to Haiti from the US. Current data from CDC states that there are almost one- half million people in the US living with AIDS. In 2006 there were 14,627 deaths from AIDS, and more than 50,000 are infected with HIV annually. In the1980s the spread of HIV infection in the US led to a high mortality rate from tuberculosis among people with dual TB+HIV infection.

It is estimated that 80 percent of TB patients in sub-Saharan Africa are infected with HIV, and tuberculosis is the leading cause of death among people with AIDS/HIV. In addition to development of dual epidemic of TB and AIDS, as mentioned above, the situation has become more dramatic, with the growing proportion of TB patients that have multi-drug resistant bacteria, MDR, and now XDR.

It is evident that a new approach is needed to manage the TB epidemics in Africa. Efforts by the WHO to implement the DOTS program in Africa during a period of more than ten years had a positive effect by making treatment available to many previously neglected patients. At the same time, although it was highly efficient in industrialized countries, implementation of this strategy in Africa was different. In addition to the above-mentioned deficiencies, even the main principle of DOTS (directly observed therapy) was not efficiently managed in most patients for the entire treatment period, and true supervision was a rare occasion in most African countries. That was in addition to inadequate treatment regimens administered to many TB patients with undetected MDR and XDR.

Although the synergistic and deadly effect of two epidemics, TB and HIV, it is now well recognized in most of the African countries, that the measures to control these epidemics were not properly coordinated. It was only recently that some attempts were made to coordinate these efforts, which included implementation of some joint laboratory services for efficient and rapid diagnosis of both infections. Again and again, this situation calls for the need of advanced diagnostic laboratories in African countries. In the meantime, in addition to the fire caused by the wars and violence, the African continent is on fire with these epidemics.

Controversies in Russia

My first encounter with tuberculosis was in 1944 when I was diagnosed with this disease. I was a third-year student at the medical school in Samarkand, an ancient city in Uzbekistan, one of the republics of the former Soviet Union. The Soviets were moving toward victory in the war with Germany, but life in Samarkand was difficult. Every morning trucks would collect bodies of those who had died in the streets. Most of these unfortunate souls died from starvation; however, no one knew how many of them had died from various diseases. This was in addition to a large number the people who received notice that their family members had been killed in the war. Therefore, tuberculosis was not the most noticeable problem, although it was known that the prevalence was very high and that many people were dying from the disease.

As medical students, we were not exempt. Typically, medical students tend to *discover* many illnesses in themselves while studying them in the textbooks or by observing their patients. I was skeptical when I began to feel sick. I had fever and night sweats, as well as a cough. I came to dread nights, because I knew I would have to change my sweat-soaked clothes and bedding. I thought I might have a reoccurrence of malaria that I had contracted from the previous summer when I worked in a rural area known to have an epidemic of malaria.

But with malaria, I had very short outbreaks of fever and chills that lasted no longer than an hour and it did not affect my daily activities. This new illness was quite different from malaria, and it had a devastating effect on my studies, especially in the mornings. Reluctantly, after I noticed some blood in my sputum in the mornings, I sought medical attention and was diagnosed with tuberculosis. An X-ray showed that I had a relatively small lesion, an infiltrate in the upper right lung. I was very depressed at this discovery, and according to the textbooks (written during the pre-antibiotic era), I anticipated that I would die soon. I was due to graduate in two years. So, I made a firm decision to confront this problem. I was determined that I would survive and that I would graduate! Many TB patients survived and recovered without any special treatment. I would be one of them!

I had an additional advantage that helped me in my recovery from tuberculosis. My father, Boris Heifets, was a highly respected physician with good connections among his colleagues in the city. They were physicians who worked in one of the largest military hospitals. Although the official distribution of the drug, streptomycin, was at least a year away, mysteriously these physicians had already obtained a small supply of the antibiotic. I had no idea how they got the drugs, but to my good fortune, I was secretly treated with streptomycin (in addition to other measures). It took some time, but I fully recovered from tuberculosis. After the war ended in 1945, I transferred to the Moscow Medical School and graduated in 1947. It appears that I was among the first patients in the world to be successfully treated with streptomycin!

This was a pivotal event in my life that prompted me to consider committing my professional life to the study of tuberculosis. Fortunately, or perhaps unfortunately, the control of my career was not in my hands, but of the ever-present restrictions and regulations that dominated life in the Soviet Union. It took many years of working in other fields of medicine before I finally became involved in tuberculosis research in 1969.

In the past it was not unusual in literature to refer to Russia as an enigmatic country. Russia is no longer an enigma, especially after the fall of the Soviet Union in 1990, neither is the current public health situation there, particularly as it relates to tuberculosis. By the same token, Russia should not be viewed as just another country with statistics showing high TB prevalence. It is much more complex than that. First of all, one should keep in mind that the ideology and style of official presentations by the Russian authorities regarding TB epidemics—as well as the tuberculosis control standards—are largely inherited from the former Soviet Union system.

This means, an accurate perception of the TB situation in Russia requires not only a critical view, but also a clear understanding of the system and political environment there. Therefore, analyses based on simple comparison of TB statistics in Russia with either industrialized or developing countries can be misleading. One peculiar element of the past system in the Soviet Union was a doctrine that tuberculosis, as a *social disease* is typical for a capitalist society but not for a socialist country like Soviet Union.

Contrary to expectations based on this hypothesis, tuberculosis was quite prevalent in the Soviet Union. To resolve the controversy, any information about tuberculosis (as well as other infectious diseases) was declared a state secret, and was often the subject of biased manipulations by the medical authorities. Therefore, any information about the past as a source to analyze the dynamics of events should be regarded with extreme caution. The current situation should also be scrutinized before considering the available information for analyses.

I worked for almost ten years at the Central Institute for Tuberculosis in Moscow before my emigration from the Soviet Union in 1978. Not only was research conducted at the Institute, but it also served as an organizational center for managing TB control in the country under the Ministry of Health. Working at the Institute gave me vast insight into the problem of tuberculosis within the Soviet Union, not only from the numerous confidential documents, but also by visiting various regions of the country during my inspection assignments.

In addition to knowing all these secrets, I was quite familiar with the extremely bureaucratic and inefficient system of controlling tuberculosis. After the break-up of the Soviet Union, the TB control system did not change significantly, with one exception: the secrets were exposed. With this experience in my background, I had sufficient reasons to be skeptical regarding the perception by Western experts of the situation in Russia.

During the last ten years, the international perception of the TB situation in Russia was very much influenced by an opinion expressed in the following phrase, "Because of Russian medical jingoism, tuberculosis and multi-drug resistant TB are a present and rapidly increasing risk to the citizens of Russia, and to all of us who live in the world and breathe its air". This phrase is a quotation from the last paragraph of the book by Lee B. Reichman and Janice Hopkins-Tanne titled, "*Timebomb*" (50).

How true was this dramatic prediction in relation to the danger to the Russian citizens and to the rest of the world? Does the TB epidemic in Russia represent a greater danger for the rest of the world than the TB epidemics in Africa, or India, or China, or in the whole world outside Russia? Conclusions set forth in this book deserve serious analyses, particularly because it may represent interest from a historical perspective, since Reichman's book was written in 1997 and published in 2002, and the outcome of current events may shed some light on the value of predictions made at that time.

The prevalence of drug-resistant TB in Russia is growing at the same rate as in other countries. Obviously, the TB epidemic in Russia is neither the only, nor the major threat to the US and other industrialized countries (see Appendix 4). Clearly, Russia represents a very small proportion of potential sources of infection in the world's pool of patients with active tuberculosis.

It is estimated that more than 2 million Russians travel every year to Western and Eastern European countries, but most are short tourist visits. With respect to the number of long-term visitors (not immigrants), Russian nationals do not represent a large number of travelers to the US and other industrialized countries compared to the number of visitors from Africa, India, Central America, and other countries with high TB prevalence. To single out Russia as a major source of TB or drug resistant TB to the rest of the world was an exaggeration.

However, it appears that predictions are correct regarding the anticipated increasing risk of Russian citizens becoming infected with the drug-resistant tubercle bacilli. Prevalence of drug-resistant TB in Russia has risen since 1997, but not for the reasons suggested by Dr. Reichman. It is not because at the time Russian medical professionals did not embrace the DOTS (Directly Observed Therapy, Short course) program that was recommended by the WHO.

In fact, despite Russia's formal acceptance of DOTS, the prevalence of TB increased during the years following Reichman's short visit to two TB institutions in Moscow ("walking through") on July 9-11 1997. Conclusions in Reichman's book were based mostly on this visit and brief conversations with some of the physicians and laboratory worker, and discussions with a few leading Russian personalities over dinners.

The book followed a traditional skillful journalistic approach to simplify the issues by dividing them into black and white. Dr. Prymak, who was the director of one of the TB institutions Reichman visited, and his facility was labeled as *bad* and the other one led by Dr. Khomenko was labeled *good*. In fact, neither of these institutions was "good," and the operation of both reflected the outdated TB control system inherited from the Soviet System. The only difference was in appearance: dilapidated structure and interior of "Prymak's institute" and freshly painted walls in the "Khomenko institute."

Neither place had up-to-date laboratory equipment, such as aerosol-contained centrifuges, and neither had modern biosafety standards. None of this had changed in 2005 when I visited both institutes. The primary distinction between the directors of the two institutions was based on rejection or acceptance of the DOTS strategy for Russia. The authors of the book did not realize that after the fall of the Soviet Union, the responsibility for managing the country's TB control program was transferred from Khomenko's Central institute to the TB institute of the Russian Federation. The newly appointed director of this institute, Dr. Prymak, suddenly found himself in the position of being responsible for the TB program inherited from the Central TB Institute.

For decades, Dr. Khomenko, a typical Soviet era official, was in charge of the program. I worked in his institute for almost ten years and travelled with him for inspection of the TB control measures outside Moscow. This position provided me the opportunity to witness implementation of all the components of the Russian TB control program, including individualized therapy instead of a standard treatment regimen, which Reichman so harshly criticized in his book.

When travelling abroad (one of the few trusted Soviet scientists that were allowed to do so) Khomenko played the role of an open-minded scientist, contrary to his actual behavior at home in the Soviet Union. He was allowed to socialize with the western colleagues (even inviting them to his hotel room for a drink of vodka) and earning the title of "old friend" by Dr. Reichman. Khomenko accepted the WHO policy (verbally) and implemented it in a small area (Ivanovo). He told me later in Paris that his acceptance of the WHO strategy did not change anything in the country but it provided substantial financial support in foreign currency to his institute (the program in Ivanovo is described below).

Prymak did not have Khomenko's diplomatic skills and became a convenient scapegoat. In fact, Prymak did not oppose the DOTS strategy in general, but only one of its components, the emphasis on microscopic sputum smear examination as the primary (and by some suggestions, the only) diagnostic tool. In his perception, the WHO suggested eliminating the existing bacteriological laboratories because Russia could not afford them, even though they had routinely provided culture isolation and drug susceptibility testing for many years. Only in this regard did he object to the attempts of WHO representatives to ignore Russia's experience in the field of TB diagnosis and further implying that Russia is no different than some developing countries in Africa.

In fact, Russians were not the only ones who criticized the DOTS strategy. There were other organizations, such as Doctors Without Borders (*Médicines Sans Frontières,* MSF) who in 2004 called for radical changes in this strategy because "sputum microscopy test—one of the cornerstones of DOTS, which developed in 1882, is becoming obsolete in the HIV era" and because "it detects only 50 percent or less of the TB patients" (51).

It is unfortunate in their zeal to mark Russia as another WHO-guided country that the WHO representatives overlooked the need for serious efforts to improve the operation of the TB laboratories with regard to biosafety and introduction of simple technologies for rapid and effective bacteriological methods, as well as for effective timely detection of patients with drug-resistant tuberculosis.

The events that occurred in Russia during the past decade have confirmed that the failure or success in dealing with the TB problem in Russia is not related to the formal acceptance of the WHO-recommended strategy, or to the choice of Russian personalities appointed by the government to run the National TB Control program.

What is the real TB situation in Russia today, and what were the historical roots, real and political?

After the collapse of the Soviet Union in 1991 and the subsequent organizational and economical chaos, Russia was severely affected by three concurrent epidemics. One was narcotic use, which resulted in high rates of crimes and subsequently growing prison population. The second epidemic was the pervasiveness of HIV/AIDS, closely associated with the wider use of injected narcotics. Thus, on this background, the tuberculosis epidemic continued to grow, particularly drug-resistant TB, which spread through both new patients and those who were previously treated.

A specific breeding ground for this deadly combination is overcrowded prisons, where many prisoners become infected with both, HIV and TB. Upon release, these ex-prisoners often settled in the same cities where they had been incarcerated and became a source of both infections to the local population. Release from prison often meant interruption of anti-TB treatment because the patients were reluctant to check into local civilian anti-TB facilities. Noncompliant patients and the inconsistent supply of anti-TB drugs contributed to the growth of drug-resistant TB epidemics in many areas.

Alcoholism, another important factor, coupled with long interruptions in treatment contributed to non-adherence to prescribed drug therapy. Despite implementation of programs labeled "Directly Observed Therapy", because of alcoholism, social misbehavior (particularly among former prisoners) the reality is that in Russia a substantial proportion of patients could not be forced to adhere to this principle, which resulted in a large proportion of patients failing treatment regimens, with or without DOTS.

Understanding the complexity of the TB situation in Russia, in addition to the prevailing political issues, require much more than either short visits by the western experts or taking at face value the official reports by the Russian authorities and the local Moscow WHO office.

The archaic public health system in Russia was inherited from that of the former Soviet Union without significant changes, including the system of TB control measures and regulations. Knowing the history of TB in Russia may produce a better understanding of the current situation.

Tuberculosis in Russia was unknown before 1860, and most of the cases described in the literature among the famous Russian artists, musicians, and aristocracy occurred while these individuals travelled to Western Europe, where in the nineteenth century approximately 25 percent of the population died from TB, and this epidemic was later labeled "The Great White Plague." At the end of the nineteenth and the beginning of the twentieth century, the situation in Russia began to change. A substantial portion of the predominantly rural population began moving to the large industrial cities whose hygienic conditions were far from perfect.

An enormous boost in the surge of TB epidemics in the country came during World War I (1914-17) and the subsequent revolution and the Civil War, which led to the country's unprecedented disastrous economic situation and mass starvation. Large masses of people were dislocated, creating a housing crisis. This TB epidemic coincided with the establishment of the new regime, the Soviet Union, and one of the priorities of dealing with this problem was the new government, along with the necessity of establishing measures to control other epidemics of infectious diseases, which were spreading across the country.

The Soviet Government established a network of Sanitary-Epidemiological Stations (SES), a pyramidal system with the Ministry of Health (as it is now called) at the top, not only to control the epidemics, but primarily a broad range of issues related to the health care system, environmental control, and working conditions. Within the new centralized government controlled administrative system, clinics and hospitals worked under supervision of the SES network. In the 1930s, an additional system to take control of tuberculosis was added.

These specialized institutions were called Tuberculosis Dispensaries. They were tasked with organizing TB control measures, including registration and monitoring of all TB patients in the area, identifying new TB patients, control of the ambulatory and hospital treatment, bacteriological and radiological diagnosis, and mass BCG vaccination. Additionally, a network of TB Research institutions was established to guide the local dispensaries and the entire anti-TB system.

As in all other areas of the Soviet Health Care system, the medical care (and partially general social care) of TB patients was provided free of charge. Did it not sound great? Just like a dream for those who would like to establish a similar health care system in the US in our time. Yes, it sounded great. Yes, it appeared great on paper, but it was not so in real life.

In reality, the Soviet Health Care System did not work. After all, it was part of the largely failed totalitarian Soviet System. One reason the whole system failed (including the anti-TB program) was extremely rigid control measures, being controlled by the Ministry of Health through multiple mandatory decrees (so-called "Prikaz") from the Minister of Health. Some Russian medical professionals defined it as a "Pyramidal System," for which many of them are still nostalgic. It was (and still is in Russia) a system that excluded any deviation of measures in different areas of the country that may have been necessary, depending on the local situation, thus reflecting mistrust of the local physicians and other medical professionals, depriving them of any creative thinking or initiative.

Given the disastrous economy, another major reason for the failure was that the TB control system in general, as well as many other programs including long-term treatment in the sanatoriums, was unrealistic. In addition, the well-known internal terror, not the least of which was government-imposed starvation in many rural areas. With the absence of anti-TB drugs at that time, tuberculosis was proclaimed a social-related disease, which supposedly should affect only the capitalist countries, and would be successfully eliminated under Socialism! Actually, there were official plans for TB elimination (what is new?). This socialistic dream did not materialize, and the prevalence of TB and death from TB continued to rise. A simple solution was found; statistics on TB and all other infectious diseases became a state secret.

The next disaster that confronted the country was the attack by Germany in 1942. The devastating effect of the war, along with the brutal internal political terror, resulted in economic disaster, which continued long after the war, and persisted till after Stalin's death in 1953. Management of the tuberculosis system continued unchanged since its establishment in the 1930s. Furthermore, information on the TB situation remained a state secret until the collapse of the Soviet Union in 1991.

Management of tuberculosis patients was quite archaic and expensive even in the 1990s and was not much different from the era before the discovery of anti-tuberculosis drugs. It often included hospitalization for one year or longer, expensive treatment in sanatoria, and application of numerous expensive and unproven non-specific therapies to ostensibly enhance the patients' general health. Selection of antibiotics for individual therapy was disorganized and depended on the availability of drugs in every locality, and often was based on a doctor's subjective preference. Confirmation of a diagnosis of tuberculosis was mostly based on X-ray findings, even in patients with no typical symptoms of TB.

As a basis for diagnosis bacteriological testing was, and still remains, technically inferior in most places. This fact, along with the general approach for TB diagnosis inherited from the past, resulted in 50 percent or less of the TB patients without bacteriological confirmation of their diagnosis. It is possible that the unknown proportion of patients among those with negative bacteriological results may have been misdiagnosed and perhaps had another illness.

Among those who did have TB without bacteriological confirmation, the status of the susceptibility or resistance of their bacteria to the administered drugs remained unknown. Absence of this information makes it impossible to select drug therapy to which the bacteria are susceptible for each patient. Unfortunately, it is also true for patients in whom diagnosis is based only on microscopic smear examination results without the bacterial culture isolation and drug susceptibility testing.

During the past fifteen years, in addition to exposure and relations with the rest of the world and under the weight of severe internal economic problems and political uncertainty, Russia has been challenged with a new era of confronting tuberculosis. Since 2003, the World Bank, USAID, Russian Ministry of Health, and many international non-government organizations have contributed millions of dollars to fight TB in Russia.

The WHO office was established in Moscow and a number of trials in a few sites have been conducted to demonstrate the advantages of the WHO strategy. Finally, the WHO had an opportunity to include Russia in the list of countries that accepted the WHO strategy and the leading role of this organization in combating TB in the world. Did it improve the situation in the country?

The first among the pilot studies aimed at promotion of the DOTS strategy was the above-mentioned project in the Ivanovo district (oblast) organized by the Central TB Institute in 1995 and financially supported by the WHO. Ivanovo is a relatively small district (population of approximately 1.2 million at that time) located 165 miles from Moscow. Dr. Khomenko, the Director of the Central TB Institute, initiated this project to demonstrate his personal acceptance of the WHO-recommended strategy. According to the CDC report (52), despite implementation of the DOTS strategy, the outcome of therapy with the WHO-recommended standard regimen in Ivanovo was defined as poor in nearly 30 percent of 514 smear-positive newly diagnosed patients during the period of 1995-1998.

All patients were subjected to the bacteriological study (culture isolation and drug susceptibility testing), which by definition were beyond the original DOTS program formulation. The results of this laboratory testing using the archaic technology (cultivation on the egg-based culture medium called Löwenstein-Jensen medium) for drug susceptibility of the patients' bacterial isolates were obtained too late to be used for any changes in the standard treatment regimen administered to patients. The results of this study indicated that prevalence of primary MDR-TB in the Ivanovo oblast increased during the DOTS implementation from 3.8

percent (7 out of 186) in 1996 to 9.4 percent (11 out of 117) in 1998.

Analyzing this data, the CDC experts recommended that in areas like Ivanovo with high prevalence of primary drug resistance, additional strategies were needed, "including rapid assessment of drug susceptibilities and use of alternative "second line" TB drugs." This statement was, in fact, recognition of the need for individualized treatment (instead of the standard treatment regimen) with selection of drugs for each patient based on drug susceptibility testing. It was not the original recommended DOTS strategy! It was worded as an *additional strategy* for patients in areas with high prevalence of drug resistance. The question is, are there many areas in Russia that don't have high prevalence of primary drug-resistance, where the original DOTS strategy (standard treatment regimen and no drug-susceptibility testing) would be successful?

The city of Orel was one of the few areas in Russia where DOTS strategy was more successful. This city, with a population of approximately 900,000, is located 200 miles from Moscow. The standard WHO-recommended treatment regimen was implemented in 1999 to treat patients with diagnosis either confirmed by microscopic smear examination and/or culture isolation, or without such confirmation. From a total of 310 civilian patients, 179 were culture-positive patients, six had MDR-TB, five had bacteria resistant to rifampin, and twenty were resistant to isoniazid.

Despite this situation, which was not much different from that in Ivanovo, the cure rates in Orel were higher than in other pilot studies in Russia, although the target of 85 percent cure rate was lower than anticipated by the WHO. It was 81 percent among the new smear-positive patients and 60 percent among the re-treated cases. More attention and focus from the medical professionals and a relatively smaller number of patients may explain why the program was more successful in Orel than in other locations. The outcome of therapy before implementation of the DOTS strategy in Orel was not reported.

The third set of pilot studies was conducted in Tomsk Oblast in Western Siberia with a population of approximately one million—half of whom lived in remote villages. There were many publications about the observations in Tomsk. In 1995-96 a clinical trial to compare the effectiveness of two treatment methods was funded by the Department for International Development in the UK. Newly diagnosed patients were divided into two groups: one (390 patients) was treated under the DOTS strategy using WHO-recommended standard treatment regimen, and the second (356 patients) was treated under the so-called Russian traditional program, which was perceived as chaotic administration of various drugs.

Results of the study (53-54) indicated that there was no difference between the two groups in regard to the terms of recovery. The treatment success among the smear-positive patients (approximately 50 percent of all patients enrolled) was only 63 percent in both treatment groups. Treatment failure was particularly high among patients who had multi-drug resistant bacteria. The conclusion of the report was that DOTS strategy is applicable to the Russian patients.

Despite introduction of the DOTS strategy in Tomsk, the cure rate among new TB patients fell from 90 percent in 1985 to 72 percent in 2000. This was interpreted mainly as a result of the growing proportion of patients with primary drug resistance, including MDR-TB. One of the studies conducted in 2001 in Tomsk analyzed 237 newly diagnosed patients who were subjected to the standardized DOTS treatment regimen. As discovered after their treatment, many of these patients had drug-resistant bacteria before therapy: 8.4 percent were MDR-TB and 34.5 percent were resistant to at least one drug. In addition, 6.3 percent of the patients developed MDR-TB during the period of therapy with the standard regimen.

The subsequent interest in the situation in Tomsk by the international organizations and groups was triggered by the growing rates of MDR-TB, particularly between 1998 and 2002: Increase from 6.5 percent to 13.7 percent among new patients and from 26.7 percent to 43.6 percent among the previously treated patients. A number of studies were conducted in Tomsk for evaluation of various approaches for treating patients with MDR and XDR. It appeared that only a small proportion of patients were identified as having non-resistant bacteria and should have been considered eligible for the WHO-recommended standard treatment regimen.

The problem was that the outdated laboratory system and technology in Tomsk, as well as in most places in

Russia, did not allow rapid detection of drug-resistance to differentiate between patients who were eligible for the DOTS standard regimen and those (with drug resistance) who should have been treated from the very beginning with an individualized treatment regimen.

Observations in all three areas of Russia described above were interpreted by the WHO representatives and by those involved in these studies as evidence of the successful implementation in Russia of the WHO-recommended DOTS program, although the program had changed and expanded its original version while preserving the term DOTS. In addition to the disputes between the Russian and WHO authorities, introduction of the DOTS strategy and the enhanced DOTS-Plus program had after all, a positive effect by making the management of TB patients more systematic, better controlled, and more cost-efficient. Nevertheless, the overall TB situation in Russia did not improve. Based on the data from the 2002 WHO report that worldwide in 2000, the treatment success in DOTS-areas was 82 percent vs. only 62 percent in non-DOTS area, and in Europe it was 77 percent vs. 72 percent. No similar data were reported in Russia.

The growing epidemic of drug-resistant TB is a major problem in Russia that was not addressed properly by the DOTS programs, primarily because of insufficient laboratory services. Adequate laboratory services would have ensured timely detection of drug-resistance in patients, and thereby allowed for alternative treatment regimens.

In September 2010, The World Bank and the WHO office located in Moscow, jointly issued a report on the current TB situation in Russia. It sounded optimistic regarding the achieved success. According to this document, one of the elements of success was an increase in the number of regions from 14 in 2003 to 83 in 2007 that adopted the WHO-recommended DOTS strategy with implementation of the standard short-course treatment regimen. It is peculiar that in one of the sub-titles of the report the term DOTS is described as *Directly Observed Treatment Strategy* with *Strategy* (for *S*) instead of *Short-course regimen* as it was in the original WHO documents.

Other achievements listed in the report are as follows: an increase to 75 percent of patients for whom the clinical manifestation of TB was confirmed by microscopic sputum smear examination; an increase of patients' compliance with the standard treatment regimen increased from 44 percent in 2004 to 75 percent implementation of surveillance of resistance to the first-line drugs, etc.

In Russia the incidence (the number of new TB patients reported annually) in the year 2000 rose to 90.7 per 100,000 population (a total of about 127,000 patients) and still remained high despite the decline to 82.6 in 2009. For comparison, the incidence of TB in the US is less than 5 per 100,000. These statistics may not be accurate, and the average data do not reflect variations among the different parts of the country and various social groups, with above-average rates among prisoners. The report does mention the problem of drug-resistant tuberculosis, but not the growing rates of this occurrence.

The report from Moscow is a typical politically correct document, praising the successful implementation of all the elements of the original DOTS program, but still fell short of compliance with the 2010 WHO updated policy. For example, there is emphasis on importance of the "access to quality sputum microscopy for case detection" as a major diagnostic tool, but there is no mention of implementation of modern methods for culture isolation and drug susceptibility testing, and nothing about the actual improvement of laboratory services!

The recommendation of the 2010 WHO (concurrently issued in Geneva) report was "to focus on enhancement of laboratory services." The US Action Plan of 2009 stated, "The laboratory plays a critical role in the diagnosis and management of drug-resistant TB." The report from Moscow indicated that laboratories at all levels were strengthened, but failed to say how and, additionally, that the laboratories were provided with 42,000 units of modern laboratory equipment. Perhaps, a large number of microscopes were among these *units*, but there were no aerosol-contained centrifuges or tools for rapid laboratory diagnosis of TB or detection of drug-resistance.

During the period between 2001 and 2007 I visited many Russian TB laboratories in Moscow, St. Petersburg, Yekaterinburg, Novosibirsk, Irkutsk, and Blagoveshchensk. I can testify from this experience, as well as from discussions with many Russian microbiologists who visited my laboratory for training, that at the time of my visits, none of the laboratories were equipped for implementation of Biosafety Level 3 (BSL-3) practices as required in the US and European countries.

None of the laboratories had an aerosol-contained centrifuge, without which the laboratory can become a source of TB infection for lab personnel and everyone in the building where the laboratory is located. It is not surprising that the prevalence of TB among Russian laboratory employees is 10 to 20 times higher than in the rest of the population. Use of *ancient* centrifuges is also an indicator of the ineffective methodology for detection of tubercle bacilli in patients' specimens. There were many other problems with safety and efficiency.

Altogether, for the most part, the Russian TB laboratory system is ineffective in identifying patients with drug-resistant tuberculosis and does not have the capacity to provide timely information needed by the physicians for effective treatment of these patients. I spoke with many individuals in the Russian Health Care administration who still believe that implementing biosafety regulations is a formal issue and, therefore, not important. They insisted that for Russia, Level 2 biosafety is sufficient.

In contrast, Russia has a cadre of the most experienced and knowledgeable microbiologists who enthusiastically perform their duties, and struggle to do their best under the most difficult limitations (very low compensation in unsafe conditions), which sadly, are often imposed for political correctness. Furthermore, authorities sometimes underestimate the role of the laboratory in prevention of drug-resistant tuberculosis that ultimately results in more efficient therapy.

My visits to several cities in Siberia as a consultant to the Euro-Asian Medical Educational Program (EMEP) of the Institute for Health Policy Analyses (director—Dr. Edward Burger) were the most educational for me. One of these visits was of particular interest. In June of 2007 Dr. Edward Burger, Dr. Donna Sweet (an expert on AIDS from University of Kansas) and I visited the city of Irkutsk near the famous Lake Baikal. Our lectures at the local medical school were well received.

Interactions with the Russian medical authorities, faculty members of the Medical School, and the local government representatives were cordial, with mutual understanding of the problems, and the incomparable famous Russian hospitality. Most of the medical facilities were of the highest modern level. Irkutsk had sufficient resources to construct and develop the most advanced diagnostic center staffed and managed by well-educated professionals, and equipped with modern imported equipment. In stark contrast was the overall management of TB.

We scheduled a visit to the oblast TB dispensary hospital, and of special interest to me was the fact that they had twelve patients with TB meningitis, which is extremely rare in adults. In my past experience as a physician, I only saw this disease in children; even a few cases of TB meningitis in a community were viewed as an indicator of a highly unsatisfactory TB situation.

The next day when we arrived at the hospital, we were told that two of the twelve patients had died overnight.

All of these patients had AIDS, which contributed to development of disseminated TB. As a result, the tubercle bacilli spread into the brain's membranes, causing meningitis. These patients had arrived at the hospital in a coma. At least four of them were recovering from both, TB and AIDS, due to the intensive and highly skillful treatment of both diseases by a female doctor working in the hospital. All of the patients were young men in their early twenties, who when posing for pictures, appeared healthy and happy.

The physicians and medical personnel were highly skilled and worked under very difficult and dangerous conditions, yet they successfully treated many patients with drug-resistant TB and AIDS. There were no problems with the supply of anti-TB and anti-viral drugs, but the environmental conditions were abysmal. At the time of our visit, there were almost three hundred TB patients in the hospital who were housed in an overcrowded dilapidated ancient building, with four-to-eight patients in small wards and others were in beds in the corridors.

Patients with drug-susceptible tuberculosis were not isolated from those with drug-resistant TB. More than half (almost 70 percent by one of the reports) of the patients in Irkutsk had drug-resistant TB. Similar conditions in hospitals were evident in other cities as well. Russian experts claim that hospitalization may be the source of drug-resistant bacteria in patients who were not previously infected. This fact confirmed, however, the concept of putting TB patients in single-bed rooms was not foremost in the mind of Russian medical professionals and administrators. Instead, to prevent the spread of drug-resistant tubercle bacilli among the TB patient, they consider less effective and inefficient ambulatory treatment during the first two to three month intensive phase of therapy.

Contrary to the opinion of some western experts, effective ambulatory treatment is not feasible in most Russian cities where the residential areas are widespread and lack public transportation and most individuals do not have personal transportation. My colleague, Dr. Michael Iseman, and I became keenly aware of this situation when we visited the city of Pervouralsk, located in the Ural Mountain region. In such places, for the majority of Russian patients, at least during the first two to three months of the intensive treatment, Directly Observed Therapy could not be implemented without hospitalization. This situation was quite different from that in Newark, NJ, and even from large cities in Russia like Moscow. Therefore, one of our recommendations to the Irkutsk authorities was to consider construction of a modern TB hospital as priority, taking into account the severe epidemics of TB, drug-resistant TB, and AIDS/HIV.

Another recommendation was to build a modern TB laboratory with proper biosafety conditions and affordable technology that would allow rapid detection of patients with drug-resistant tuberculosis. Timely diagnosis of patients with drug-resistant tubercle bacilli is hampered by the use of the Löwenstein–

Jensen (L-J) method which was introduced almost one hundred years ago. Turnaround time for reporting drug-susceptibility test results by this method is three to six months or longer.

Not only is this technology outdated and inappropriate, but the whole Soviet-style laboratory service system was not designed to help physicians in a timely diagnosis of TB or in identifying patients with drug-resistant tubercle bacilli. At the time of our visit, ten laboratories and forty so-called "seeding stations" handled the TB laboratory services in Irkutsk Oblast. The raw specimens were processed in these stations, and the inoculated L-J slants were then forwarded to the laboratories, where identification of the growing organism—and for some—drug susceptibility tests (with first-line drugs only) were performed.

For final evaluation, the cultures were sent to the Oblast Dispensary laboratory in Irkutsk. Obviously, this multiple-step operation increases the already lengthy turnaround time of the laboratory reports. The reports containing the drug-susceptibility/resistance pattern of patients' isolates were generated too late for the results to be useful to the physician's decision. We recommended replacing this system with direct submission of the specimens to well-equipped laboratories.

To date, none of our recommendations have been implemented. The Irkutsk region is now considered by the local TB administration as one of the regions in Russia with the highest prevalence of TB+HIV patients (512 new patients in 2009 alone) and with 72 percent of TB patients with drug-resistant tubercle bacilli.

The recovery rate is very low (51-65 percent among TB patients). Meanwhile, the local administration is reluctant to implement any of our recommendations, or to address the issues of biosafety. Instead, their focus is on the basic research and implementation of sophisticated molecular laboratory methods.

Fortunately, there are some entities in Russia (such as laboratories in Moscow, Novosibirsk TB Institute, and many organizations in Yekaterinburg of Sverdlovsk Oblast) where the local authorities are committed to proper changes in TB control measures, particularly focusing on improvement of laboratory services. Especially impressive was a project developed in 2001-02 for the huge Sverdlovsk Oblast located around the Ural Mountains.

With support from the above-mentioned EMEP organization, there were four leading microbiologists from Yekaterinburg who were trained in my laboratory in Denver. Subsequently, in consultation with the local medical authorities, we analyzed the TB situation in the Sverdlovsk Oblast and developed a project focused on centralization of the laboratory services. The project was presented at the World Congress of Tuberculosis in Washington, DC in 2002. The plan was to close down small laboratories and the *seeding stations* and organize direct delivery of the specimens to five large TB laboratories to be properly equipped, and therefore, provide test results within the shortest possible turnaround time.

However, it was only in Tallinn and Tartu, cities in Estonia where I saw modern laboratory environment with superior services. Development of these laboratories is an indication that it is possible to have highly-rated TB laboratory services in areas with limited resources, and still have enthusiastic professional leadership. This is a prime example for Russia, where the epidemic of drug-resistant TB is skyrocketing. It is much worse than indicated in official reports (see below), because these reports document only the prevalence of MDR-TB cases, while other forms of drug-resistance are not included. In some areas of Russia, the majority of TB patients are those that have various types of drug-resistant tubercle bacilli other than MDR.

Emergence of the MDR-TB epidemics developed in Russia (see Appendix 5) despite introduction of the DOTS strategy. Perhaps the growing prevalence of MDR-TB was the result of the so-called amplification phenomenon, where the standard treatment regimen was universally applied to all patients including those with undetected resistant bacteria due to ineffective testing.

At the time of Dr. Reichman's visit in 1997, the TB situation and the TB control system in Russia were bad, but it has since become much worse. Acceptance of the WHO-recommended DOTS program, viewed by Dr. Reichman and many other experts as a solution to Russian problems, did not improve the situation. The number of TB patients reported annually may have slightly declined over time, however, a substantial proportion of drug-resistant tuberculosis cases appeared. Although introduction of the DOTS program possibly had a positive effect on the country's outdated philosophy of the medical professionals, the main principles of the original WHO-recommended strategy were presented too late and could not prevent the growing prevalence of drug-resistant tuberculosis. Standardized WHO-recommended treatment regimen did not work for most patients with drug resistant bacteria.

The original DOTS strategy emphasis on sputum smear examination as the main diagnostic tool, along with the other neglected bacteriological methods, resulted in insufficient and incomplete detection of new TB patients in the communities. No significant efforts were made to improve the laboratory services for timely and effective detection of drug-resistance. With outdated laboratory technology (such as the egg-based L-J culture medium) approximately 50 percent of all patients did not receive bacteriological confirmation of their diagnosis and no information regarding susceptibility of their bacteria to the anti-TB drugs they received.

Even under the new WHO recommendations on the importance of the laboratory services in the era of MDR and XDR epidemics, the situation has not changed. In order to be "politically correct" the Russian documents issued by the local WHO office have modified this recommendation to accommodate the original DOTS strategy. One example is a remarkable phrase in the document: "...introduction, and support of the enhanced laboratory services through high quality *microscopic examination*." In addition, some

Russian scientific groups are trying to introduce highly sophisticated molecular methods that are not applicable in the routine practice of the diagnostic laboratories. In the meantime, no serious efforts are being made to introduce simple modern cultural methods for reasonable and timely detection of drug-resistance, and no efforts are being made to enact proper biosafety standards.

Only modern TB laboratories with direct centralized services are capable of providing bacteriological confirmation of TB diagnoses and drug susceptibility testing in a timely manner to greater than 50 percent of new patients. In other words, there will be no effective system in Russia to provide individualized treatment for patients with drug-resistant bacteria. Without dramatic changes in laboratory services the epidemic of drug-resistant TB will continue to grow unabated.

The circumstances in Russia can be defined as a process of recycling from regular TB into an epidemic of drug-resistant infection, with a substantial proportion of cases with difficult-to-treat multi-drug resistant (MDR-TB) and extensively drug resistant (XDR-TB) tuberculosis.

The predominant indicator regarding the general public health situation in Russia is reflected in the substantial decline in the population: from 148 million in 1990 to 143 million in 2010, with predictions of further decline to 111 million in 2050, due to the increasing mortality and declining birth rates. The primary cause of the increase in mortality (annual rate of 15 per 1,000) is attributed to alcoholism, but the tuberculosis epidemic, especially in combination with HIV/AIDS, may become one of the contributing factors to the accelerating mortality rates in the near future.

New Hopes in India

Meeting Durai at the graduation party in New York appeared to be a turning point in Martha's life. Living all her life in a relatively small southern city of Mobile, Alabama, Martha did not have a chance to meet any men from exotic places like India. She just graduated from the University in Mobile and started thinking about the future, professionally and personally. Her cousin, Emma, graduated at the same time and invited Martha to a graduation party at the American University in New York. Martha was in awe of the big city, and was very much impressed with the diversity of people she met in New York.

After the party, Martha continued meeting Emma's Indian friends during her almost four-week stay in New York. The men were graduates from the most prestigious universities in India, and, as such, became desirable candidates for some American companies. They were sophisticated intellectuals who achieved high positions in their employment within a short period of time. Martha began spending a lot of time with Durai, a very attractive young man in his late twenties, and the inevitable happened—they fell in love.

A formal wedding ceremony was held in Martha's hometown, but a large traditional Indian wedding was held in an area called Tamil Nadu in Southern India, where Durai's parents lived. Spending two months in India represented an opportunity for Martha to discover a different world. Martha had no trouble adapting to the hot and humid climate of India, after all she was from the Deep South. Martha was eager to learn about the sophisticated cultural heritage of the Indian people, as she visited a number of historic temples, and enjoyed the hospitality of Durai's many relatives.

Two observations had a particularly shocking effect on Martha. One was the contrast in living conditions between the affluent and luxurious cities and the extreme poverty in some villages. The other was the fact that many people had tuberculosis. Some of them, in the cities, received appropriate treatment in the local medical facilities, but many others (mostly in rural areas) were not even diagnosed with tuberculosis. Having TB was often a stigma, especially among the people with a lower level of culture and education.

Therefore, it was not polite to call attention to anyone who was diagnosed with this illness. At the same time, it was known that some people, even Durai's extended family, had TB. It was not unusual to hear people coughing while spitting on the ground. Martha, a future medical student, was quite aware the danger this abhorrent behavior represented, but she was helpless in limiting her contact with those around her. After returning to the US, Martha and Durai settled in New York.

However, their wedded bliss was interrupted two months later when Martha was diagnosed with a latent form of tuberculosis. Fortunately for Martha, she did not have active disease, but the diagnostic skin test was positive indicating that she had a latent form (non-active TB infection) requiring preventive anti-TB treatment for many months until her skin test became negative.

The Republic of India is not only the world's most populous country (approximately 1.2 billion; 70 percent of which live in rural areas), but also a country with the highest prevalence of tuberculosis in the world. From a total of 9.4 million new cases in the world in 2009, 1.98 million were in India. One should keep in mind, that not so long ago the TB situation in India was much more severe than it is today (see Appendix 6). It is important to stress that most of the patients were diagnosed on the basis of direct microscopic examination of their sputa. Due to very limited application of methods that are more sensitive than microscopy, only about 50 percent of all TB patients in the communities were detected.

The medical professionals in this country recognize this problem and are currently pursuing implementation of culture isolation, drug susceptibility testing, and molecular methods for better detection of TB patients in general, and in particular, those with drug-resistant tubercle bacilli. Therefore, in the near future, one can anticipate a change in statistics showing an increase in the number of detected and reported cases of tuberculosis.

According to the official report, the prevalence of MDR-TB in new patients (so-called primary MDR resistance) was only 3 percent, which is more than 50,000 cases, already a significant source of MDR bacteria to potentially infect people in some communities. In addition, MDR was detected in 14-17 percent of patients who had previously been unsuccessfully treated (so-called retreated cases). Unfortunately, these estimates do not reflect the actual magnitude of the problem, because in 2009 only 6,000 patients were suspected of having MDR and subjected to the appropriate laboratory testing; one thousand of them were diagnosed with MDR.

This alone suggests that the prevalence of MDR-TB in India could be much higher than officially reported—an official estimate is 131,000 MDR-TB cases, based on a survey in only two states—if more patients were subjected to appropriate laboratory testing beyond sputum microscopy. It is also estimated that approximately 50,000 detectable MDR cases emerge annually in India, and it can be assumed that the prevalence of MDR-TB is significant. The actual magnitude of this problem can be better assessed in the future, after broad implementation of drug susceptibility testing, rather than the current estimate obtained from surveys conducted in selected areas.

India has a reputation as a country with the strongest governmental commitment to address the problem of tuberculosis. Therefore, along with the fact that the country has many highly qualified medical professionals and specialized institutions, there is room for optimistic predictions for the future, despite the possible negative impact of the growing rates of HIV/AIDS. It was estimated that in 2007 there were 2.3 million individuals living with HIV/AIDS, and the proportion of TB patients co-infected with HIV ranged between 5 to 7 percent. It is assumed by the report that the TB epidemic in this country is driven by non-HIV cases. Perhaps — but not yet! Combined measures against both TB and HIV are among the future strategic plans.

India was one of the countries that accepted the DOTS strategy at its initial introduction by the WHO. Implementation of measures associated with this program was definitely beneficial in a country that did not have a defined national program. Acceptance of the new WHO Stop TB Strategy in 2006-2007 by Indian officials helped to further improve the situation. The statistical data quoted above illustrates this improvement. In addition, adherence to the WHO recommendations placed the country on the list of *politically correct* entities that helped in receiving necessary financial support from the World Bank and other sources.

The question is whether strict adherence to these programs and their limitations will help to achieve further progress. The following questions remain: (1) How is detection of TB going to proceed with patients with smear-negative specimens? The unidentified number is perhaps close to 2 million, based on the well-known fact that microscopic smear examination—the main tool under the initial WHO guidelines—can only identify half of the TB patients, (2) How will patients with drug-resistant TB (including those with MDR-TB) be identified? We must keep in mind that the number of such cases is perhaps much greater than the number reported by selective testing for this phenomenon of only 6,000 patients.

Fortunately, the leadership in this country and most of the medical professionals do understand the complexity of the situation. On one hand, they fully accepted the new WHO Strategy, which includes "good quality diagnosis through sputum microscopy". In this program, the strategic vision for the year 2015 is formulated "to achieve 85 percent cure rate and 70 percent case detection of new smear-positive cases" (*Global WHO Plan: Stop TB Strategy, Geneva, 2006*).

The guidelines for MDR-TB management in the *Revised National Tuberculosis Control Program (RNTCP)* suggested implementation of the so-called DOTS-Plus services, beginning in ten states, and subsequently expanding to other states. In other words, it means the broad use of culture isolation, drug susceptibility testing of the patients' isolates, and individual selection of drugs for treatment based on this testing instead of using the standard treatment regimen. Even so, it is the "*S*" in the DOTS acronym for "Short course Standard Regimen," which is necessary for political correctness. The important part of this program, regardless of political correctness, is the wording in the following statement: "The vision is to have a network of RNTCP accredited quality assured state level Intermediate Reference laboratories (IRLs), at least one in each large state, providing culture and Drug Susceptibility services..."

In addition, the existing four National Reference Laboratories would supervise the operation and training of IRLs personnel. Development of a system of comprehensive laboratory testing puts India among the countries with hope for effective prevention of epidemics of MDR-TB and XDR-TB. Of course, there are inevitable obstacles on this reasonable path, including financial problems, optimal design of the laboratories, and choice of the most appropriate technologies, including both cultural and molecular methods.

In addition to conventional cultivation methods, many of the new technologies are available in a few advanced institutions covering testing of a limited number of patients. These technologies are considered for future implementation with the purpose of expediting the laboratory reports, so that the physician would be able to make adjustments in the selection of the drugs for therapy in each patient as soon as possible. Evaluation and validation of these methods is conducted as joint projects with the Foundation for Innovate and New Diagnostics (FIND).

Among these technologies are automated liquid medium systems and various molecular methods for rapid laboratory TB diagnosis and rapid detection of drug resistance. Evaluation of these and other new methods, promoted by various manufacturers, will not only address their efficiency, but also their practical application, including cost-efficiency and the overall cost of a large-scale implementation.

Although development of some of these methods represents significant progress, the practical introduction of these methods throughout the country may face dilemmas—mostly related to very high cost. One example is the GeneXpert MTB/RIF technology, which is recommended by FIND and is already available in India in limited experimental settings. This automated system was developed by the Cepheid Company and has recently become the subject of collaborative research sponsored by FIND and performed by a large group of institutions in several countries. It was highly publicized in the 2010 September issue of *The New England Journal of Medicine* and by the media.

Within two hours the system can detect the presence of tubercle bacilli in a sputum specimen and determines whether the bacteria in the specimen are resistant to rifampin, the most important anti-TB drug (as a marker for MDR). The method is much more sensitive than the microscopy test in detecting the bacteria in sputum specimens, which, as mentioned before, is positive in less than 50 percent of TB patients, while nearly half of all new patients remain undetected. The new molecular test developed by Cepheid is said to be capable of detecting the presence of tubercle bacilli in sputum specimens in up to 85 percent of all new TB patients. This system is advertised as a potential for replacing the microscopy test with this procedure. One instrument is capable of only running between one and four specimens at a time, which is approximately about one hundred specimens per week, or less than 5,200 specimens per year of intensive use of the instrument.

According to the official report, in 2009 the microscopy of the sputum smears was used for examination of 7. 2 million suspected TB patients. Can this country afford to have more than one thousand Cepheid instruments to replace (or to supplement) microscopy, keeping in mind the cost of each machine is $30,000 (or $20,000 with a possible discount) and supplies at $40.00 or at least $20.00 per test? Perhaps, it may have only very limited and selective application, but not as an overall solution for rapid and complete detection of MDR-TB cases in this country. Perhaps, other molecular methods, less expensive than the Cepheid procedure and more comprehensive detection of resistance should be considered, for not only to rifampin, but to other drugs as well.

One of the important features of the Cepheid system is that it can be used in a physician's office and does not require a laboratory setting! In other words, this system is introduced not as a supplement to the laboratory protocols, but instead of in-laboratory testing. Implementation of Cepheid or any other molecular system alone does not resolve the problem of efficient search for patients with MDR-TB (and XDR-TB) in a community. An alternative is the above-mentioned plan for development of a network of laboratories for culture isolation and drug susceptibility testing.

India's medical authorities will have to make choices for the most optimal combination of conventional and molecular methods in fully developed laboratories *vs.* limited implementation of the Cepheid or other similar systems outside of the laboratory network.

The New White Plague Can Be Prevented

There were three most important documents addressing the future of tuberculosis at the global and the US national levels:

"The Global Plan to Stop TB, 2006-2015" launched in 2006 by the World Health Organization (WHO):

1. "Multidrug and extensively drug resistant TB (M/XDR-TB), 2010 Global Report on Surveillance and Response", also issued by the WHO
2. "Plan to combat extensively drug-resistant tuberculosis, recommendations of the Federal Tuberculosis Task Force," published in 2009 by CDC (54)

The first of these documents, the Global WHO Plan of 2006 consisted of six *Millennium Development Goals* (MDG), and each of them contained a number of specific targets. One of these targets was formulated as "halt and begin to reverse the incidence of TB by 2015," which means to achieve a situation in the world when the number of annually reported new TB cases start to decline. Another remarkable target is: "by 2050: eliminate TB as a public health problem (one case per million population)" (*Global WHO Plan: New Stop TB Strategy, Geneva, 2006*).

Only the distant future will reveal how realistic these rather optimistic predictions were. Some of the current events and statistics may support such an optimistic view, but other facts are causing serious doubts on the possible future trends of the TB epidemics. Particularly alarming is a phrase in the WHO documents explaining how the proposed goals of the program would be achieved, "The core of this strategy is DOTS, the TB control approach launched by WHO in 1995." Does this mean implementation of the DOTS strategy in its original form introduced in 1995? If asked, the authors of the document would probably respond negatively, because the current DOTS strategy has been significantly modified from the original.

There are no critical comments in the document regarding elements of the original DOTS that cannot work in areas of high prevalence of primary MDR and other forms of drug resistance. It is not clear whether the document permits following the original DOTS version or suggests application of the recently upgraded

DOTS version. Lack of clarity on this issue may *tempt* some local leaders to choose the easier method using the original DOTS. That means the possibility that a patient may be treated with drugs (under the standard regimen) to which his/her bacteria are resistant. Also, it allows flexibility of limiting the diagnosis of TB to sputum microscopy (without cultivation), which means incomplete detection of TB patients in the communities and no detection of patients having drug-resistant tubercle bacilli.

More than four years have passed since the WHO issued the 2006-2015 Plan, and it is reasonable to question the changes and progress that took place during this period of time. The optimistic view of the future can be derived from some facts presented in the aforementioned second WHO document issued in March of 2010. Among these facts are the following: since 1995 nearly thirty-six (or forty-nine) million patients around the world were treated under DOTS-based services; in 2008, an estimated 62 percent of new smear-positive patients were treated under DOTS, and the treatment success among *these* patients reached 86 percent in thirteen out of 27 high-burden TB countries.

These results are indicative of the potential of treatment results under DOTS strategy, but do not reflect the overall actual situation in these thirteen countries, because nearly half of the patients with negative smear microscopy results were neglected and not included in the overall calculation of the outcome of therapy. Also, the results in fourteen other high-burden countries remained unknown.

The same data, being a source for optimistic prediction, may also be viewed as a source of concern, doubts, and questions. One concern is that only patients with sputum smears positive on microscopy were the focus, which means that those patients with negative test results (more than 50 percent of all patients) were neglected. In other words, only approximately 30 percent of *all* patients were treated in thirteen out of 27 countries. This means that 70 percent of all patients including those in thirteen successful countries did not receive any anti-TB treatment in 2008. What about the remaining fourteen high-burden countries? That was the real situation during 2008, the year considered the most successful for DOTS implementation.

Another obstacle to the success in TB control is the increasing epidemics of HIV/AIDS, particularly in Africa, Asia, Russia, and in other parts of the world. The HIV infection greatly affects immunity rendering one highly vulnerable to TB. After years of debates among the health care providers, the national programs in many countries encompass combined measures to control both TB and HIV. Nevertheless, the prevalence of HIV/AIDS is growing in many parts of the world. For example, in 2007 about one million cases of TB (from a total of more than nine million new cases in the world) were associated with HIV infection. It is estimated that at least 30 percent of the HIV-infected individuals in the world also have TB, and TB is one of the predominant causes of death among the HIV-infected.

In hindsight even more doubts about the success of future plans to defeat TB and achieve the above mentioned goals for 2015 and 2050 can be derived from the main point of the 2010 WHO report, which is emergence of epidemics of MDR-TB (and XDR-TB) as a new major challenge in many countries. Around 500,000 new cases of MDR-TB emerge each year in the world (estimated 440,000 in 2008). These numbers do not include the unknown situation in most of the African countries, and an estimate on the MDR burden is available only for four among them: South Africa, Nigeria, Democratic Republic of the Congo, and Ethiopia.

Other 27 countries classified in the WHO report as high-burden MDR include the following: India, China, Bangladesh, Indonesia, Viet Nam, Pakistan, Myanmar, Philippines, Bulgaria, and fourteen countries of the former Soviet Republics (Armenia, Azerbaijan, Belarus, Estonia, Georgia, Kazakhstan, Kyrgyzstan, Latvia, Lithuania, Russia, Moldova, Tajikistan, Ukraine, Uzbekistan). These 27 countries account for 85 percent of all known MDR-TB patients, with India, China, Russia, South Africa, and Bangladesh having the largest numbers.

The MDR statistics do not include larger numbers in either the 27 high-burden countrics, or other countries that have patients with other than MDR types of drug-resistance that may affect the outcome of therapy with the standardized treatment regimen. For example, as presented in previous chapters, in some Russian cities up to 70 percent of patients had various types of drug-resistant tubercle bacilli. Application of the standardized treatment regimen to all patients is highly problematic without identifying those who have drug-resistant bacteria, particularly in high-burden MDR countries.

For years, debates among the TB experts were focused on whether or not it is possible to achieve any positive results in treating MDR patients with the WHO-recommended standardized treatment regimen. It is well known now that treatment of the MDR-TB patients with the WHO-recommended standardized treatment regimen is not effective. Eventually, it was shown that the possibility of successful treatment of the MDR-TB patients exists if the so-called second-line drugs are used instead of the standard regimen, and the drugs are administered for a long period of treatment.

One should keep in mind that the probability of death from TB among the MDR-TB patients—particularly among those who are defined as XDR-TB—may reach the level of the past during the pre-antibiotic era. Dr. Michael Iseman, my colleague at National Jewish Health in Denver, demonstrated that it is possible to cure MDR-TB patients with an individualized regimen that included drugs selected on the basis of drug susceptibility testing performed in our laboratory.

On a larger scale, to the surprise of many skeptics, my good friend Dr. Paul Farmer and his group in Lima, Peru, observed 78 percent cure in a group of almost one hundred patients that had bacteria at least resistant to rifampin and isoniazid and defined as MDR-TB. According to the 2010 WHO report, with proper management, the treatment success of the MDR-TB cases can reach 60 percent. Again, the patients in Lima were treated with drugs selected on the basis of drug-susceptibility testing of the patient's bacteria. That was if and when a patient with MDR was identified!

The problem is that, as was the case in Peru, it may take several months for the lab results to indicate the status of the patient's bacteria (susceptible or resistant to various drugs). When I visited Lima, I observed that patients were suspected of having MDR only if, after at least three months, they did not respond to therapy with any improvement in their condition of treatment with the standard regimen (including rifampin and isoniazid).

Then there was an attempt to isolate the culture of tubercle bacilli by cultivation on the egg-based medium, a technology that takes up to eight weeks. If the culture was isolated, it was sent from Lima, Peru to the State Laboratory in Boston for drug susceptibility testing with mostly the first-line drugs. For additional testing with second-line drugs the culture is subsequently sent from Boston to our laboratory in Denver.

Altogether, it takes many months for the data on the drug-resistance pattern (including confirmation of MDR) to become available to a physician in Peru, it may take up to a year from the time the patient was diagnosed with TB until the potentially successful treatment with the second-line drugs is started. In the meantime, the patients continued to suffer and to spread drug-resistant tubercle bacilli throughout the community.

There is a high probability of treatment failure of the standardized treatment regimen in patients that have undetected drug-resistant bacteria when information on their drug susceptibility pattern is not available at the beginning of therapy. There is also the possibility that the partially resistant bacteria may become MDR. As a result, patients treated ineffectively continue to infect others with drug-resistant strains of tubercle bacilli. The only solution to the problem in selection of drugs for treatment is to obtain information on the drug susceptibility/resistance pattern of the patient's bacteria in a timely manner.

The enormous problem is the cost of the management of the MDR-TB patients, including the cost of second-line drugs and hospitalization considered necessary for these patients. According to the WHO report, about 1.3 million of MDR/XDR-TB cases will have to be treated between 2010 and 2015 in 27 high MDR-TB burden countries only, the cost of which is estimated to be $16.2 billion over a period of six years, which is sixteen-fold more than what is available. This estimate does not include the MDR-TB and XDR-TB cases in countries other than those 27 listed above.

Additionally, one should keep in mind, that besides MDR-TB patients, there are unknown numbers of unreported patients that have tubercle bacilli with drug-resistance other than MDR who would most likely respond poorly to the standard treatment regimen. It seems that the situation is like an avalanche. The alternative is that if countries, indeed the world, do not properly address the epidemics of MDR-TB and

XDR-TB now, they will face an insurmountable financial burden in the future. Treatment of MDR-TB patients is highly cost-efficient and diminishing epidemics will have a significant impact on future economy of many countries. The first important step in this direction is the least expensive elements—establishment of an efficient laboratory system to provide comprehensive and timely identification of patients with drug-resistant tuberculosis in the communities.

There were statements and complaints by the medical leadership in a number of developing countries about the difference in standards recommended by the WHO and other international organizations for handling TB in developing countries *vs.* those that exist in industrialized countries. The major effort to address this issue was made in the two above-mentioned WHO documents. In reality, it is not just recognition of the needs for proper management of TB in developing countries, but the financial support of these activities.

So far, this support, in significant part (at least 14 percent of cost), depended on contributions from international organizations and groups, as well as on donations from industrialized countries. The only way to fill the aforementioned gap between the funds available from these sources and those needed, is to make the issue of TB control a financially significant part of each country's budget, as it is in most of the industrialized countries. It is expensive, but the alternative for not doing will be much more costly!

The international funding to cover the cost of any part of the program is definitely unrealistic. No such funds are available! Perhaps, therefore, a full-scale program to prevent an epidemic of incurable tuberculosis can be feasible in only some countries at the time, and it should be primarily based on the national resources if available, with focused only on additional support from outside.

The question is, which country or countries will become pioneer(s) to initiate a comprehensive program based on provisions of the national budget? It is important that the international organizations and groups focus attention and resources on such a country to support development of a model of success in prevention of the epidemics of drug-resistant tuberculosis.

To date, the document introduced in 2009 by the Federal Tuberculosis Task Force *Plan to Combat Extensively Drug-Resistant Tuberculosis* is the best plan to address the issues of drug-resistant TB. It can and should be used as a model for countries other than the US. This plan is the most recent update from the previously published documents a work that started after the US faced an unprecedented TB resurgence, predominantly the emergence of MDR-TB cases from 1985-1992.

The emphasis of this comprehensive document is on the sixty-seven unresolved specific problems in the areas of diagnostic laboratories, epidemiology, infection control, legal issues, education, and research, needed to be addressed for effective prevention of epidemics of drug-resistant TB, particularly MDR-TB and XDR-TB. Detailed steps of action are formulated to address each of the sixty-seven problems identified in the document, with a note as to whether any of the recommendations may have either domestic or international implications.

The first fifteen problems listed in the document are related to the Diagnostic Laboratory, which indicates recognition that the laboratory plays an important role in addressing the TB situation today. However, laboratories do face problems. Even in the US some TB laboratories are not capable of identifying XDR, and in many international laboratories the personnel need additional training. Laboratories in many countries don't have sufficient up-to-date capabilities for complete testing, and send the patients' specimens to other countries, which delays the results for timely treatment management of the patients.

There is an important difference from the dominant international approach in that the US document never mentioned the *affordability* of any of the proposed recommendations. They must be implemented at any cost! In other words, similar to the US, the approach in other countries would become possible under conditions at a much higher cost than the current financial commitment. With the current economic and political situation in most countries having high TB and MDR-TB prevalence, these problems are not yet perceived as high priorities in comparison to other national problems; often there is no vision of the rapidly approaching disaster in either medical or economic terms of an epidemic of incurable TB.

The prevailing attitude in some countries and international organizations is to do *something* within the limits of affordability. It has never worked before (such as limiting the activity to only patients diagnosed by the direct microscopic smear examination), which resulted in the spread of drug-resistant tubercle bacilli from patients not diagnosed under such conditions with either positive or negative results of the microscopic examination. Implementation of a magic bullet type solution, such as a rapid molecular method intended for use instead of establishing a laboratory may increase (compared with smear microscopy) the number of patients diagnosed with TB, but it would not prevent the spread of drug-resistant bacteria.

Measures to prevent epidemics of drug-resistant TB include a number of elements well defined in both national and international programs, including the DOTS (in recent updated definitions). Implementation of the whole program may be very costly, but it can be practical to start with an element, which is often neglected as described above — organization of a system for efficient laboratory diagnosis, including identifying patients who are excreting drug-resistant tubercle bacilli.

Laboratories—The Ultimate Weapon

The growing epidemics of drug-resistant tuberculosis, especially MDR-TB and XDR-TB around the world, have recently triggered a new understanding of the urgent need to identify patients with drug-resistant tubercle bacilli in the communities. It has become evident that without timely detection and proper treatment of these patients nothing can be done to prevent further spread of the epidemics caused by the dangerous drug-resistant tubercle bacilli. Therefore, rapid identification of patients with drug-resistant tuberculosis has become the highest priority.

A sensational publication in 2010 September issue of *The New England Journal of Medicine* appeared to be a solution of all TB problems. It was introduction of an automated system called *GeneXpert MTB/RIF* by the Cepheid Company (See chapters "Recycling of the

White Plague" and "Hopes in India.") The Cepheid system can detect tubercle bacilli in a patient's sputum within two hours, and also determine whether these bacteria are susceptible to or resistant to rifampin, resistance to which is a likely indicator that it is MDR. It is said that this system is highly sensitive and able to identify the presence of tubercle bacilli in sputum of approximately 85 percent of all TB patients (*vs.* 50 percent by microscopy, yet still less effective than by cultivation).

The major advantage of this molecular system is that it can be used out of the laboratory setting, such as in the physician's office, which opportunity may be welcomed by some (or many) physicians. This development is endorsed by the WHO and other organizations, and heralded by the media as the major solution of the TB problem in the world. The system would be very useful in remote areas of the world that do not and will not have full-scale TB laboratory services in the near future.

This system is already being sold around the world. Without a doubt, the system will become even more popular if the manufacturer develops additional options, such as testing more specimens at the same time, testing for HIV along with TB, expanding the test to drugs other than rifampin, introducing the possibility of using solar energy in areas that don't have stable electrical power, and making the system more affordable.

In addition to the intensive marketing of the Cepheid system, so far not much attention has been given to the fact that resistance to rifampin is only a part of the bigger picture. Depending on the results obtained by the Cepheid system, without proper broader laboratory testing, to which drugs the bacteria are susceptible, would remain unknown, thereby providing physicians with various treatment options. Also, it is not capable of identifying patients with XDR.

The system has a limited capacity for testing only four specimens at a time and it is very expensive. Each instrument costs at least $20,000 (or in anticipation of a large sale $17,000) in addition to $20.00 or $40.00 for supplies per each specimen. It is highly questionable whether implementation of this currently available system (in large numbers) in sites with thousands of patients to be tested would be less expensive than development of full-scale TB laboratories.

In the most recent analyses (55) the major advantage of the *GeneXpert MTB/RIF* system, its potential for application in low-income countries is questioned not only due to the high cost, but also to the environmental limitations, such as stable electricity, maintenance, etc. The authors even suggest that this system should be used only in large hospitals and the major emphasis in TB diagnosis in such countries should be on high quality microscopy. What about rapid detection of drug-resistance and what about having TB laboratories in large hospitals?

Currently, in most of the industrialized countries and in many developing countries the answer to whether patients' specimens contain tubercle bacilli and whether they are drug-resistant can be obtained within 24 hours or even in few hours from the modern

TB laboratories equipped with both conventional and rapid molecular methods. For example, a technology developed by *Hain Lifescience* and available in TB laboratories in more than seventy countries not only allows determination of the presence of tubercle bacilli in the patient's specimen within four to five hours, but also whether they are resistant or susceptible to rifampin, isoniazid, quinolones, and injectable drugs.

In other words, it determines whether the patient has MDR or XDR, which is subsequently confirmed by conventional laboratory methods. Within 24 hours it also provides the physician with information regarding drugs to which the bacteria are still susceptible, which is necessary for choosing agents for a justified treatment regimen.

Often, the Cepheid system is perceived as a panacea. In this regard, one should remember lessons of past history in many fields of medicine; without becoming a part of the complex measures, any single development has never resolved major problems. It is especially true for tuberculosis, mainly because this disease requires a very long period of therapy, with more than one drug at the same time.

Even such great developments as discovery of tuberculosis bacilli, the development of the BCG vaccine, or the beginning of the era of anti-tuberculosis antibiotics with the discovery of streptomycin, did not change the situation alone. Currently, the emphasis by the major international and national policy-making organizations to control TB epidemics is made up of complex measures, among which the proper laboratory services are taking priority.

Nevertheless, due to extensive marketing efforts, the Cepheid system became an attraction for policy-making medical administrators for implementation not only in areas without proper laboratory services, but also in countries where laboratories can provide the above described full scale testing including the rapid molecular methods such as from *Hain Lifescience*. The reasoning for having the Cepheid system outside the laboratories, in close proximity to the physician's office, is to have results available within two hours that can be used to make a speedy decision as to how to treat the patient. The specimen will be subsequently sent to the laboratory (where such laboratories exist) based on the result of such preliminary testing. There are several problems with this algorithm:

1. The processing of the whole specimen in the Cepheid system results in killing the tubercle bacilli, and another specimen must be collected to send to the laboratory, which is not always possible.
2. If the result of testing by Cepheid system shows that the bacteria are susceptible to rifampin, the standardized treatment regimen would be administered, but it is well known that in a number of cases, susceptibility to rifampin does not exclude resistance to isoniazid, and the standard regimen containing isoniazid may not be effective in such cases.

3. Without isolating the culture, which can be done only in the laboratory, tuberculosis may not be diagnosed in nearly 30 percent of patients, which may happen if the second specimen is not collected for testing in the laboratory.
4. Discovering that the patient's bacteria are resistant to rifampin does not give the physician directions to which other drugs may be selected for treatment. To answer this question in areas that don't have properly equipped laboratories, another specimen must be collected and shipped out for drug-susceptibility testing, which may have an extended turnaround time before a lab report is received. In the meantime, the MDR patients will be treated empirically using inappropriately selected treatment regimen and may spread the dangerous MDR bacteria to others, if the treatment regimen is ineffective.

Introduction of the Cepheid system occurred following the general recognition of the problem of the epidemics of drug-resistant tuberculosis and comprehensive new programs were recently developed on the international and national level.

In response to the problem of the MDR and XDR epidemics, in 2009 the Centers for Disease Control and Prevention (CDC) published the above quoted document entitled *Plan to Combat Extensively Drug-Resistant Tuberculosis, Recommendations by the Federal Tuberculosis Task Force.*

One of the most impressive elements of this plan is shown in two statements:

1. "The laboratory plays a critical role in the diagnosis and management of drug-resistant TB. The test results must be available in a time frame that allows clinicians to make prompt patient management decisions" and
2. "The prompt and correct diagnosis of drug-susceptible and drug-resistant TB is the cornerstone of effective TB control."

The contrast between previous neglect and present recognition of the role of laboratories and in identifying patients with drug-resistant tuberculosis is amazing! In 1990, the American Thoracic Society joined with the Centers for Disease Control and published an official statement on TB: "Given the low prevalence of drug-resistant *M. tuberculosis* in most parts of the United States, the cost of routine testing of all initial isolates is difficult to justify."

In other words, at that time, for the sake of cost efficiency, performing drug-susceptibility testing with the cultures of tubercle bacilli isolated from patients (and even performing isolation/cultivation of tubercle bacilli) was discouraged. At the time the price of such testing was less than $50.00 per patient, and the statement was made in spite of outbreaks of multi-drug resistant tuberculosis that had already begun in the US.

The change in attitude toward the necessity of laboratory testing was now recognized at the international level as well. The 1997 the World Health Organization (WHO) guidelines stated, "Susceptibility testing is not recommended in all new cases of smear-positive pulmonary tuberculosis… since it is not practical, it is expensive, and it is useless". In 2010, WHO issued the above quoted document titled, "Multidrug and Extensively Drug Resistant TB (M/XDR-TB), Global Report on Surveillance and Response", which refers to the laboratory services by stating, "The laboratory plays a central role in patient care and surveillance…"

Although both document, from the CDC and the WHO, bring to the forefront the role of laboratory services today, there are some important differences in the details. In the US document, the goal is to get prompt results regarding each patient, while at the international level there is still emphasis on surveillance for estimation of the general situation in a country or specific area.

The WHO document stated that one of the critical steps in controlling MDR-TB is establishing reference laboratories to supervise drug-susceptibility testing (DST) performance in smaller laboratories. In 2008 only half of the 27 countries with high MDR-TB rates had contemporary laboratory diagnostics. Often, in some countries there was only one laboratory with the capability to culture tubercle bacilli from patients specimens and to perform the drug-susceptibility test, mostly with only few first line TB drugs.

According to the WHO Report, under the "Global Laboratory Initiative" a multi-national project called

EXPAND-TB was started with $87 million dedicated to laboratory upgrades (with new and rapid diagnostics) in 15 high MDR-TB burden and 12 other countries over a period of five years. This substantial investment may become a good starting point for a real solution to the problem of timely diagnosis of the MDR-TB patients in the communities.

At least one example of increasing laboratory services under the EXPAND-TB program raises hope that the process may be headed in the right direction. This example is the recent joint efforts by the Ethiopian Health and Nutrition Research Institute (EHNRI), Foundation for Innovative New Diagnostics (FIND) and other partners to establish at least two modern TB laboratories in Addis-Ababa, Ethiopia.

These laboratories are designed for Biosafety Level 3 practices, to incorporate modern cultivation method in a liquid medium system, and to implement one of the molecular methods for rapid direct detection of tubercle bacilli in the patients' specimens, as well as to determine resistance to rifampin as a marker of MDR (*Line Probe Assay Technology*).

This development illustrates the feasibility of having laboratories for rapid detection of TB in general and MDR in particular in a resource-limited country. It is not clear whether the TB laboratories in Addis-Ababa are serving as reference laboratories only, or represent a system of services for testing specimens delivered directly from patients. The outcome of this progress is not yet known. It is estimated that there were 5200 cases of MDR-TB in Ethiopia in 2008, but so far only 130 of them were detected and reported.

In 2008, the situation in countries with high MDR-TB burden demonstrated the contrast between the numbers of estimated and actual notified cases of MDR-TB. There was an estimated total of 380,000 cases of MDR-TB in these 27 countries, which is approximately 85 percent of all such cases in the world, but only 23,216 of them were actually reported (and properly treated). In 2008, nearly 50 percent of all MDR-TB cases in the world, or approximately 200,000 MDR-TB cases, were in China and India, but only a small proportion of them were reported (and properly treated).

Overall, the drug susceptibility testing for both new and retreated TB patients is rare, and it is far from systematic activity in high-burden MDR-TB countries. Among these 27 countries, only a few are without an official National Reference Laboratories (NRL) as required by the WHO, but it is evident that having an NRL is not a guarantee for proper detection of the MDR-TB cases in a given country.

With or without NRL, identification of patients with MDR-TB is at record low level, even in the 27 countries that are the focus of attention by the WHO and the world medical community. Without being identified, these patients are not subjected to proper therapy and remain a source of infection with drug-resistant tubercle bacilli in the communities. So far only one percent, which is a very small proportion (as suggested in the WHO report) of the identified

MDR-TB patients around the world in 2008, received treatment with expensive second-line drugs selected on the basis of drug-susceptibility testing of their bacteria.

Undoubtedly, the most effective and reliable way to determine which of the available drugs to which the patient's tubercle bacilli are susceptible or resistant is to perform appropriate testing in a specialized laboratory. There is a stark contrast in this regard between industrialized nations (USA, Japan, and most of Europe) and developing countries. Unfortunately, there is still a widely held opinion that many among the developing countries cannot afford full-scale TB laboratories.

Consequently, a search for possible alternatives continued at the national and international levels. As addressed above and in some of the previous chapters, the predominant scenario in the past (and currently remains in many situations) was to have a network of microscopy stations. It is now universally recognized that TB diagnosis by microscopy alone not only misses nearly half of all new patients, but also does not detect those who harbor drug-resistant tubercle bacilli. With the growing epidemics of drug-resistant tuberculosis, the quest for a solution was inevitable. One of the most recent suggestions discussed above is the introduction by the Cepheid Company of an automated system GeneXpert MTB/RIF.

One of the problems of implementation of the Cepheid system in areas that don't have laboratories may become the excuse for some decision-making medical administrators to not develop TB laboratories at all. While the Cepheid system is an important revolutionary development, it should not replace the laboratories, but rather complement other methods of identifying drug susceptibility patterns, and be implemented only when needed and when affordable.

There were many other suggestions for an alternative to TB laboratories. Some of them appear almost anecdotal. For example, there is a serious suggestion of using a special breed of rats (Gambian pouched rats, or *Cricetomys gambianus*) found in Zambia that after proper training were able to detect by sniffing, which of the sputum specimens presented to them contained tubercle bacilli. But to date, there are no claims that the rats can detect resistance to rifampin.

There are many widely spread misconceptions regarding the optimal system of TB laboratory services and even about the proper capability of the modern TB laboratory. Therefore, it is not surprising that among the 60 problems identified in this document the US plans to combat XDR, the need for education regarding proper laboratory capabilities in a broad range of health-care providers and policy-makers is listed as number one.

It is often not the opinion of laboratory professionals, but rather the policy-makers and administrators that organization of a modern TB laboratory is a very sophisticated task and it is very expensive. Insufficient information in many countries resulted in opposition and fear of implementing Biosafety Level 3 (BSL-3) practices in TB laboratories.

Another misconception that existed in the US in the past was inherited from the three-level system of the TB laboratory services. Under this system, patients' specimens were transferred from the lower level labs to a higher-level lab, which delayed reporting the results. Currently, in the US submission of specimens directly to state laboratories is encouraged. Most of the state TB laboratories are equipped with modern instrumentation and have properly trained qualified personnel.

Unfortunately, the outdated multi–level system is being introduced in some countries today, without learning a lesson from the experience in the US. The idea of de-centralization of TB laboratory services, still promoted by the WHO, was introduced along with the original DOTS program under which the emphasis was on microscopy smear examination at the network of microscopy stations to be supervised by a National Reference Laboratory, with very limited application of culture isolation and drug-susceptibility testing.

As mentioned above, today, in the era of MDR-TB and XDR-TB epidemics, the needs are different, and a broad application of cultivation of tubercle bacilli is inevitable. It is impractical—logistically and economically—to establish a network of small laboratories to address this problem. It would be much more cost-effective to have large well-equipped laboratories with professionally trained personnel to handle a large number of specimens delivered directly to such laboratories. Besides economic benefits, a system of direct services would allow inclusion of one rapid methods into the lab protocol and would result in an expedited report on rapid identification of MDR-TB and XDR-TB patients. Only an expert calculation in each country or area-specific situation can show the financial advantages of the direct centralized TB laboratory services *vs.* de-centralization.

The number of such large laboratories and the size of each laboratory for an area or a country, as well as the necessary equipment, should be estimated on the anticipated number of specimens to be received. Based on experience in a few laboratories practicing direct centralized services (particularly in Yekaterinburg, Russia, Hong Kong, Estonia, and in South Africa), the optimal size is by a design for processing between 500 and 700 raw specimens every day. At the time of my visits in the 1990s and 2002-2003, these laboratories were performing culture isolation on various media, and drug susceptibility testing on each specimen smear examination.

Perhaps today, these or similar laboratories will need to include some rapid molecular tests into operational protocol for expedited detection of MDR. There are such molecular methods—much less expensive than the above-described Cepheid system—that are capable of detecting resistance to a number of drugs (not only to rifampin) that constitutes a probability that the patient has MDR or XDR. The results are available within 48 hours. An important difference from the Cepheid system is that such technology (for example, from the Hain Life Science Company) can only be used in the modern TB laboratory that have Biosafety Level-3 environment.

It is now universally recognized that TB laboratories should play an essential role in combating the epidemics of drug-resistant tuberculosis, but such declaration is only the first step toward actual identification of patients with MDR-TB and XDR-TB in the communities. So far, in most parts of the world, it is only a goal, but not yet a reality. Establishment of modern TB laboratories with direct centralized services (not just reference laboratories) can turn the tide in effective identification of patients with drug-resistant tuberculosis to be subjected to proper therapy.

Conclusion

Conflicting optimistic and pessimistic opinions can be found in the literature on the future trends of the TB epidemics, particularly those caused by drug-resistant tubercle bacilli. Often these conflicting opinions and interpretations were derived from the same facts and from the same official documents analyzing the situation and featuring plans to combat TB.

As presented in the chapter "The New White Plague Can Be Prevented," optimistic predictions dominate the official international/WHO documents, particularly with regard to the projection of reversing the incidence of TB in 2015 and to eliminate TB as a public health problem by 2050. The facts that can be derived from the same WHO documents do not support this optimism. This is especially true in dealing with the epidemics of multi-drug resistant tuberculosis (MDR-TB).

In these documents it is recognized that timely identification of patients with drug-resistant TB is essential for proper treatment and prevention of the spread of drug-resistant tubercle bacilli. Moreover, the role of laboratories in this process is declared as the key element in prevention of MDR epidemics. At the same time, these documents do not go much beyond the general declarations, and no effective and realistic specifics are suggested for enforcing the elevated role of the TB laboratories.

Particularly optimistic is the recent review from CDC. The authors emphasized the success of the DOTS strategy during the last fifteen years: "…treating nearly 49 million persons and curing 41 million with TB" (56) which, according to this review, resulted in saving six million lives. The article stresses the need for development of new rapid (molecular) methods for detection of drug resistance of tubercle bacilli in patients' specimens.

Unfortunately, it does not address the issue of organization of the laboratory services in developing countries with description of the US past experience, which is a lesson to learn for other countries, still struggling with the dilemmas surrounding the issue of rational laboratory services. In fact, this experience, which ended with the establishment of centralized services in the US instead of previous three-level system, is a good argument for being optimistic about the TB future trends in the US.

Optimistic predictions regarding the world situation are usually based on some statistical data, as presented in the chapter "The New White Plague Can Be Prevented." Since 2004 the number of people affected by TB has slightly declined and the general attitude of the world community changed from complete neglect in the past to better understanding of the problem and of the need for many measures introduced worldwide. At the same time, one should keep in mind that there are growing numbers of patients with drug-resistant TB, including MDR-TB and XDR-TB, along with somehow improving statistics regarding the total numbers of TB patients. Today TB still kills more people than AIDS, malaria, and leprosy combined, and every 20 seconds, TB takes the life of another human being in the world.

In hindsight of all the above-described controversies, all of the optimistic and pessimistic predictions, the three main questions to be asked regarding the future TB situation are:

1. Is it possible to prevent the new white plague in principle?
2. Under what conditions is it possible?
3. Is it realistic to anticipate implementation of necessary measures that would prevent emergence of the new white plague worldwide in our time?

The answer to the first of these questions is definitely yes. The answer to the second question is that it is possible under the conditions of full implementation of the requirements listed in the international (WHO) and US national documents—quoted above—plus fundamental upgrade of the laboratory services beyond the general statements made in the International documents.

The critical point is the answer to the third question. The situation is problematic. As quoted above from the WHO report only the cost of treating MDR-TB patients in 27 countries with high-burden MDR-TB within the next six years is estimated at $16.2 billion, which is about 16 times more than is available, as stated in the report. More billions of dollars are needed to address other issues in these and other countries, including measures to prevent the spread of epidemics of all forms of drug-resistant tuberculosis.

According to the most recent information in 2010 the total annual expenses for TB control in 118 countries has grown to $4.1 billion, which is still short by $2.1 billion from the funding requirements set up by the "Global Plan to Stop TB 2006-2015." (57) An encouraging fact is that 86 percent of the expenses were provided from the national government budgets of these 118 developing countries and only 14 percent from external contributions.

The most important among many necessary TB-control measures is the need for fundamental changes in the laboratory services and estimation of the cost of such changes, which were not specified beyond the general declarations in the international WHO programs. After all, the reality of implementation the well-known necessary measures depends on financial support, much greater than what is currently considered to be available by the international community.

In other words, tremendous efforts to recognize the situation worldwide and in each country are needed as the first step in direction of achieving the goal of preventing the epidemics of incurable TB. What is also needed is not only recognition of the dangerous situation, but appropriate actions and financial responsibilities at both, local and international levels.

In the meantime, a specter will continue to haunt the world—the specter of the new white plague, the specter of epidemics of incurable tuberculosis.

Appendix 1: Glossary of Terms and Acronyms Used in This Book

WHO: World Health Organization

CDC: Center for Disease Control and Prevention

IUTLD: International Union Against Tuberculosis and Lung Diseases

DOTS: Directly Observed Therapy, Short-course, or WHO TB Strategy

ATS: American Thoracic Society

Mycobacterium tuberculosis, or tubercle bacilli: bacteria causing tuberculosis

Infectiousness, or contagiousness: conditions of the TB patient that made him a source of infection to others

Latent tuberculosis, or LTBI (latent tuberculosis infection): a person is infected with tubercle bacilli, but does not have active disease and is not infectious for others

Active tuberculosis, or TB: an active disease with damage to various tissues and organs caused by tubercle bacilli; TB patients may have different levels of infectiousness, the highest among those with TB lesions in lungs (pulmonary tuberculosis),

Anti-tuberculosis drugs (antibiotics):

- first-line drugs: rifampin (RMP), isoniazid (INH), streptomycin (SM), ethambutol (EMB), pyrazinamide (PZA)
- second-line drugs: amikacin (AK), kanamycin (KM), capreomycin (CM), ethionamide (ETA), quinolones (moxifloxacin, ofloxacin, levofloxacin), linezolid, cycloserine (CS), clofazimine (CF)

WHO–recommended standard treatment regimen:

- intensive phase: simultaneous administration of INH, RMP, PZA, and EMB (or SM) during a period of two (or three) months
- continuation phase: INH and RMP for a period of 4-to-6 months

Drug-resistance: status of a patient, when any part of his/her population of tubercle bacilli is resistant to anti-tuberculosis drugs

Acquired drug-resistance: resistance of the tubercle bacilli developed during the period of therapy as a result of inappropriate treatment with antibiotics, non-adherence of the patient to the prescribed treatment regimen, insufficient dosing of the drugs and/or period of treatment

Primary drug-resistance: patient has drug-resistant tubercle bacilli from the very beginning, before any treatment, as a result of infection with such bacteria from another patient

Multi-drug resistance (MDR): resistance of tubercle bacilli to main anti-TB drugs, INH and RMP, with or without being resistant to other antibiotics; MDR can be primary or acquired

Extensive drug resistance (XDR): resistance not only to RMP and INH, but also to quinolones and any of the three injectable drugs—AK, KM, CM

Smear-positive (specimen or patient): tubercle bacilli are detected under microscopic examination of a smear made from patient's sputum, which is indicative that the specimen contains more than 10,000 bacteria per ml

Smear-negative (specimen or patient): no tubercle bacilli detected under microscopic examination of a smear made from the patient specimen; it does not exclude that the patient has tuberculosis, but it may be an indication that the specimen contains less than 10,000 bacteria per 1 ml; around 50 percent of all TB patients belong to this category,

Appendix 2: Main Statistical Data on TB in the World and in the US

According to the 2009 WHO report, the prevalence of tuberculosis in 2008 was estimated at about 9.4 million new cases globally resulting in a rate of 139 per 100,000 population. The most recent WHO report of 2010 indicates that in 2008 there were an estimated 440,000 cases of multidrug-resistant tuberculosis (MDR-TB) resulting in the death of 150,000 patients. MDR-TB cases have been reported in more than fifty countries, and the WHO considered 27 of them as "high MDR burden countries". For example, in seven areas of the former Soviet Union, the proportion of MDR-TB in new cases ranged between 12 and 27 percent, and more than 50 percent of the previously treated cases.

At the beginning of 2010, fifty-eight countries have reported emergence of extensively drug-resistant TB (XDR-TB). It is estimated that by 2015 we will face nearly 1.6 million new cases of drug-resistant TB annually, and it is hard to predict, what proportion of them will represent MDR-TB and XDR-TB cases.

In the US, about 12,000 to 14,000 new cases of TB (and 500 to 700 deaths) have been reported annually (11,540 in 2009 and 11,182 in 2010), which does not sound very alarming compared to the statistics in other countries. A substantial number of patients with drug-resistant tuberculosis were detected in the US among the newly diagnosed and previously treated patients: 2,927 MDR and forty-nine XDR cases during the period from 1993 to 2006. In 2007 alone, 107 MDR patients were reported.

Appendix 3: Statistical Data on TB in Africa

In 2005 the incidence of new TB cases reached an average of 343 per 100,000 populations, with the highest rates, above average and highest in the world, in countries of sub-Saharan area. The rates of new TB cases continued to grow, and in 2007, the rate of new cases became 363 per 100,000 reflecting 2.9 million of patients. In addition, there are growing numbers of patients with drug-resistant TB. In 2007, South Africa was the first country where an outbreak of tuberculosis caused by extensively drug-resistant tubercle bacilli (XDR-TB) was reported. These XDR bacteria evolved from MDR because of inadequate management of patients with MDR, and could possibly signal the emergence of incurable tuberculosis.

According to the 2010 WHO report, it is estimated that there were 69,000 new cases of MDR-TB reported (based on mathematical modeling) in 2008, and also a number of outbreaks of XDR-TB in some African countries. While only about 10 percent of the world population leave in Africa, more than 33 percent of the world deaths from tuberculosis occurring in African countries. The growing HIV epidemic is a major contributing factor to the TB epidemics, and more than 30 percent of HIF-infected adults die from tuberculosis.

Appendix 4: TB in Russia in Comparison with Other Countries

Between 100,000 and 150,000 new TB cases were reported annually in Russia during the last decade. These numbers should be compared with a total of 9.4 million new active TB cases reported worldwide in 2009. Russia is listed by the WHO among twenty to twenty-two countries with the highest burden of TB in the world, because the incidence rate (number of new cases annually) was greater than 100 per 100,000. Most TB cases in the world are found in Southeast Asian (50 percent) and African (30 percent) regions. Therefore, assessment of Russia's role in the world's TB epidemic requires comparison between the incidents of TB in

Russia with those in other countries, particularly in India (between 1.6-2.4 million new cases), China (1.0-1.6 million), and South Africa (0.38-0.55 million).

Appendix 5: MDR-TB in Russia

According to the 2010 WHO (Geneva) report, frequency of only MDR-TB in newly diagnosed Russian patients reached high levels in several districts (oblasts) of Russia:

- Murmansk–28.3 percent
- Pskov–27.3 percent
- Arkhangelsk–23.8 percent
- Ivanovo–20.0 percent
- Kaliningrad–19.3 percent
- Belgorod–19.2 percent
- Mary–16.1 percent
- Donetsk–16.0 percent

It is much higher in previously treated patients who return for re-treatment, for example, in the following areas:

- Archangelsk–58.85 percent
- Belgorod–51.6 percent
- Ivanovo–57.7 percent
- Pskov–50.0 percent
- Tomsk–53.6 percent

A similar situation (with rates ranging from 50 to 61 percent among those retreated) also occurred in regions of other former Republics of Soviet Russia, in particular, Moldova, Kazakhstan, Latvia, Estonia, Lithuania, Armenia, Azerbaijan, and Georgia.

Appendix 6: TB in India

The incidence of TB was 568 new cases per 100,000 in 1990, a decrease to 185 per 100,000 in 2009. The death rate from tuberculosis declined from 41 per 100,000 in 1990 down to 24 per 100,000 in 2009 (still, almost 3,000 people died from TB). Over the years, a large proportion of TB patients did not have access to treatment, and it wasn't until 2009 that 1.53 million TB patients were treated. Approximately 400,000 have not yet been treated. The 2010 Indian Ministry of Health Report of 2010 stressed that in 2009 nearly 70 percent of TB patients (perhaps it meant smear-positive new patients) were detected with a cure rate of 85 percent of smear-positive patients.

References

1 Speaker A. 2011 (Interview).
2 Young A. The Atlanta Journal Constitution. 2008.
3 World Health Organization. Tuberculosis and Air Travel: Guidelines for Prevention and Control. 3rd ed2008.
4 MMWR. Extensively Drug-Resistnat Tuberculosis —- United States, 1993-2006. 2007(11):250-3.
5 Gandy S. USA Today. 2007.
6 Gandy S. 9 News.com; 2007.
7 Daniels R. (Interview) 2009.
8 MMWR. Federal Air Travel Restrictions for Public Health Purposes —- United States, June 2007-May 2008. 2008;57:1008-12.
9 Associated Press. London, Tuberculosis Capital of Western Europe. USA Today. 2010.
10 Brock TD. Robert Koch: A Life in Medicine and Bacteriology: ASM Presss; 1998.

11 Heifets L. Metchnikoff›s recollections of Robert Koch. Tubercle. [Biography Historical Article]. 1982 Jun;63(2):139-41.
12 Heifets L. Centennial of Metchnikoff›s Discovery. Journal of Reticuloendothelial Society. 1982;31:381-91.
13 Kaufmann SH, Mittrucker HW. Vaccination against tuberculosis: current status and future promise. Seminars in respiratory and critical care medicine. 2004 Jun;25(3):345-52.
14 Fanning A, Fitzgerald M. In: Raviglione MC, editor. Tuberculosis: Informa Health Care USA, Inc.; 2006. p. 541-54.
15 Hesseling AC, Behr, M.A. In: Schaaf H.S., Zumla, A., editors. Tuberculosis: Saunders Elsevier; 2009. p. 759-70.
16 Rhines C. The Relationship of Soil Protozoa to Tubercle Bacilli. J Bacteriol. 1935 Apr;29(4):369-81.
17 Waksman S. *Time Magazine*, 1949; ***Proc. Soc. Exper. Med., 1944.***
18 Hinshaw HV, Feldman, W.H. Proc Mayo Clinics. 1945;20:313-8.
19 Hinshaw HV, Feldman, W.H. JAMA. 1946;132:778-82.
20 British Medical Research Council. Brit Med J. 1948;2:769-82.
21 Auerbacher I. Finding Dr. Schatz: iUniverse; 2006.
22 Dubos R, Dubos, J. The White Plague. Boston: Little, Brown and Company; 1952.
23 Ryan F. The Forgotten Plague. Boston: Little, Brown and Company; 1992.

24 Daniels TM. The Captain of Death: The Story of Tuberculosis:. University Press; 1997.
25 Chretien J. The Illustrated History of a Disease: Hauts de France; 1998.
26 Brosh A, et. al. PNAS. 2002;99:3684-9.
27 Wingerson L. Archeology, 2009.
28 Bates JB, Stead, W.W. Medical Clinics in N. America,1993.
29 Dheda K, Migliori GB. The global rise of extensively drug-resistant tuberculosis: is the time to bring back sanatoria now overdue? Lancet. 2012 Feb 25;379(9817):773-5.
30 Lerner BH. Revisiting the death of Eleanor Roosevelt: was the diagnosis of tuberculosis missed? Int J Tuberc Lung Dis. 2001 Dec;5(12):1080-5.
31 Abrams J. Blazing the Tuberculosis Trail. Colorado Historical Society; 1990.
32 Jereb J, Abalak R, Castro KG. Sem Resp Clin Care Med. 2004;25(3):255-69.
33 Raviglione MC. Sem Resp Clin Care Med. 1997;18(5):419-29.
34 Pablos-Mendez A, editor. Antituberculosis Drug Resistance in the World. World Health Organization; 1998; Geneva.
35 World Health Organization. Guidelines for the Management of Drug-Resistant Tuberculosis. 1997.
36 Kimberling ME. Int J Tuberc Lung Dis. 1999;3(5):451-3.
37 Portaels F. Int J Tuberc Lung Dis. 1999;3(7):582-8.

38 Laserson KF. Int J Tuberc Lung Dis. 1999;3(suppl. 1):S118-S9.

39 Heifets L. Recycling of the White Plague: Prescription for Disaster: Keynote Lecture. In: Tuberculosis, The Real Millennium Bug. The International Colloquium. Antwerp: Kluwer Academic Publishers; 2000.

40 Schlossberg D. Tuberculosis and Nontuberculous Mycobacterial Infections. In: Espinal MA, Raviglione MC, editors. Tuberculosis and Nontuberculous Mycobacterial Infections, 2011.

41 American Thoracic Society. Amer Rev Respir Dis. 1990;142(3):725-35.

42 Tenover FC, Crawford JT, Huebner RE, Geiter LJ, Horsburgh CR, Jr., Good RC. The resurgence of tuberculosis: is your laboratory ready? Journal of Clinical Microbiology. 1993 Apr;31(4):767-70.

43 Crofton J, Chaulet P, Maher D, Grosset J, Harris W, Horne N, et al. Guidelines for the Management of Drug-Resistant Tuberculosis. Geneva: World Health Organization; 1997.

44 World Health Organization. Multidrug and Extensively Drug-Resistant TB (M/XDR-TB), 2010.

45 Farmer P, Bayona J, Becerra M, Furin J, Henry C, Hiatt H, et al. The dilemma of MDR-TB in the global era. The international journal of Tuberculosis and Lung Disease. [Comment]. 1998, Nov;2(11):869-76.

46 Voelker RA. The World in Medicine: Ebola with Wings. JAMA. 1998;280(14):1216.

47 Bates JH, Stead WW. The history of tuberculosis as a global epidemic. The Medical Clinics of North America. [Historical Article]. 1993 Nov;77(6):1205-17.

48 Pillay M, Sturm W. Evolution of the Extensively Drug-Resistant F15/LAM4/KZN Strain of *Mycobacterium tuberculosis* in Kwa-Zulu-Natal. Clin Infect Dis. 2007;45:1409-14.

49 Raviglione MC, Zignol M. Global MDR and XDR-TB, Situation and Trends, 2010.

50 Reichman LB, Hopkins-Tanne J. Timebomb: The Global Epidemic of Multi-Drug Resistant Tuberculosis. New York: McGraw Hill; 2002.

51 Ahmad K. MSF Tuberculosis Report Criticises DOTS Strategy. The Lancet Infectious Diseases. 2004;4(12):719.

52 Centers for Disease Control. Primary Multidrug-Resistant Tuberculosis — Ivanovo Oblast, Russia, 1999. MMWR. 1999;48(30):661-3.

53 Mawer C, Ignatenko N, Wares D, Strelis A, Golubchikova V, Yanova G, et al. Comparison of the effectiveness of WHO short-course chemotherapy and standard Russian antituberculous regimens in Tomsk, Western Siberia, Lancet, 2001, August 11:358:445-449.

54.Centers for Disease Control. Plan to Combat Extensively Drug-Resistant Tuberculosis Recommendations of the Federal Tuberculosis Task Force. MMWR. 2009;48(RR03):1-43.

55 Trebucq A, Enarson DA, Chiang CY, Van Deun A, Harries Ad, Boillot F, et al. Xpert(R) MTB/RIF for

national tuberculosis programmes in low-income countries: when, where and how? The International Journal of Tuberculosis and Lung Disease. 2011 Dec; 15(12):1567-72.

56 Castro KG, Lobue P. Bridging Implementation, Knowledge, and Ambition Gaps to Eliminate Tuberculosis in the United States and Globally. Emerg Infect Dis. 2011;17(3).

57 World Health Organization. Global Tuberculosis Control: A Short Update to the 2009 Report. Geneva 2009.

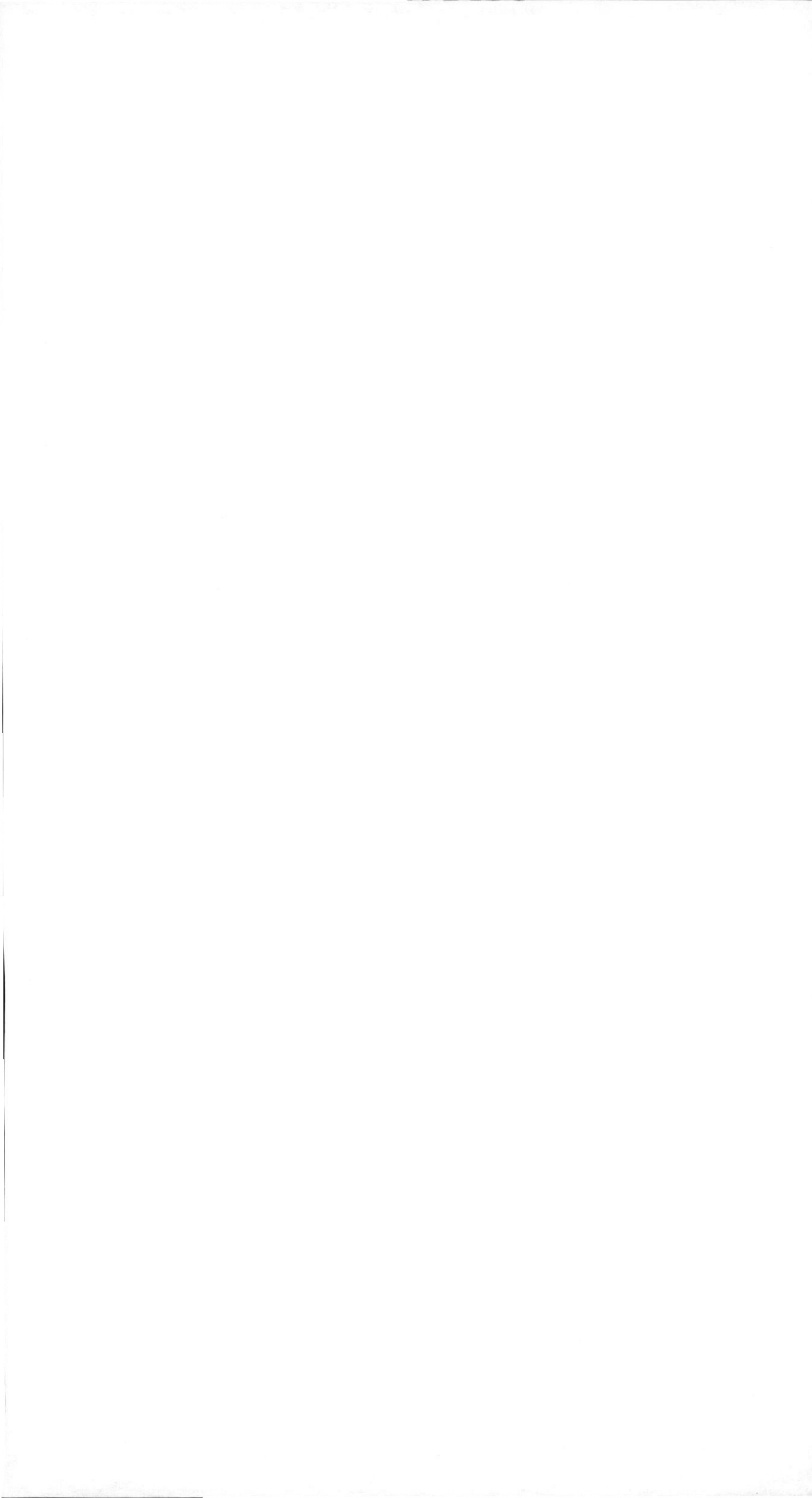